Have You Met My Grief?

*Life in The Aftermath of Loss
and Navigating A New Normal*

Jodie Atkinson

First published by Busybird Publishing 2020

Copyright © 2020 Jodie Atkinson

ISBN
Print: 978-1-922465-42-9
Ebook: 978-1-922465-43-6

This work is copyright. Apart from any use permitted under the *Copyright Act 1968*, no part of this publication may be reproduced, stored in a retrieval system or transmitted in any form or by any means, electronic, mechanical, photocopying, recording or otherwise, without the prior written permission of Jodie Atkinson

Cover Image: Kev Howlett
Cover design: Busybird Publishing
Layout and typesetting: Busybird Publishing
Author photo: Rylie Young

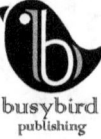

Busybird Publishing
2/118 Para Road
Montmorency, Victoria
Australia 3094

To my husband, best friend and the love of my life, Craig.

'A heart is not judged by how much you love; but by how much you are loved by others'.

~ L. Frank Baum ~

Contents

Introduction	i
1. 37 Days	1
2. Grief – The New Companion	15
3. Grief, the Thief	35
4. When Grief Just Takes Over	53
5. Supporting Someone Who Is Grieving	69
6. New Existence, New Life, New Identity	93
Final Thoughts	111
Author Q&A	115
Acknowledgements	121
About the Author	125
Resources	129
Connect with the Author	131

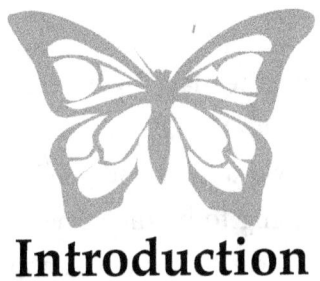

Introduction

I will never forget the day my whole world completely changed – Tuesday 7 May 2019.

The man I loved was told he had pancreatic cancer.

Life was never going to be the same again. Suddenly, we were plunged into a world of medical appointments, cancer information, limited treatment options and living with a stage IV metastatic cancer diagnosis with a short-term prognosis.

Faced with the reality that Craig was terminally ill, we were running on survival mode. How did we get here, how in the hell were we going to do this, and how would we manage our family? … And underneath every moment of doing what we needed to do, was the scary harsh reality he would not recover, knowing the day would arrive when he would not be here with me …

And just 37 days later, I lost the love of my life.

But let me rewind a bit and give you a look into what my world was like before that day.

As a personal trainer and health coach, I was running my health and fitness business and Craig was exploring new employment opportunities as he had only recently left a 25-year career in hospitality.

We were looking forward to a new chapter in our lives, one where we could enjoy our weekends together and bid farewell to nightshift and rotating rosters. We had so much to look forward to. My sons (Craig and I met when the boys were around 6 and 4 years old) were now young men and had their independence, so we were free to explore this exciting new stage.

Our days consisted of him taking our dog for a 5km walk every morning before doing some odd jobs around the house and me instructing different fitness classes and personal training sessions with clients. We enjoyed watching movies and going out for dinner. We were healthy, active, enjoying walks in nature, at the beach, working out together at home and taking the occasional holiday that involved hikes. We loved exploring new places and having an adventure that also involved our love of good food and just immersing ourselves in the experience of being in a new place with so much on offer. Tasmania was a special and favourite destination for both of us, and we travelled there on two occasions.

In particular, we loved hikes up and around Cradle Mountain, exploring Hobart – Mt Wellington, and the Salamanca Market. We thoroughly enjoyed our dining experience at Frogmore Creek on his 50th birthday, and have fond memories of the Gordon River Cruise and wandering our way around Wineglass Bay, which we experienced on our first trip.

We enjoyed visiting my parents in Victoria and Craig's family at their shack on the Spencer Gulf. We had a great group of friends, and we were excited about having more time to spend with them, enjoying weekends away, doing dinners and evenings out with them, now that Craig was more available. We had ideas for home improvements, and all the things you talk about doing if/when you have the time. We had plans. We had dreams.

Our lives were what you'd consider normal and happy. Like everybody else, we had our challenges and triumphs. But, generally, life was pretty good.

Why Am I Writing This Book Right Now?

When I was searching for grief support, I was looking for absolutely anything that made sense to me, to understand how I was feeling. I wanted to know that what I was going through, was within some range of 'normal'. See, I needed to know other people felt like I did, because that meant I wasn't losing my mind and I was not 'alone'. I needed to be reassured that I was not going crazy. I had never experienced such foreign feelings and emotions before, I was anxious, fragile and crying all the time. I was on an emotional roller coaster, I felt numb and my head felt foggy and it was incredibly distressing. I felt all different things at different times. Above all, I just felt broken and helpless.

I was so unprepared for what grief would feel like when I lost my husband, and how it would show up in my life. I have lost family members, friends and significant people in my life, so no stranger to what I understood to be grief. I just remember it feeling different. I felt those losses deeply. I was so sad, cried a lot and I missed them.

But this time it was big. I had no idea what I was about to experience. I completely underestimated the impact that Craig's death would have on my entire existence.

No one told me I would have severe panic attacks.

No one told me I would lose my sense of identity.

No one said I would experience anxiety and feel fragile.

Nothing prepared me for the deep painful ache I felt.

I had no warning I was going to feel vulnerable.

No one told me I would feel fearful to leave my house.

I had no idea that I would wonder if I was losing my mind or going crazy for feeling the things I felt and the thoughts I had surging around my brain.

I did not know that grief can creep into every single fibre of your being, make your body feel like a warzone and just fuck with your whole life!

And I probably would not have thought that was possible had they told me, either.

I knew I could not deal with this on my own. I did not trust that I had the ability to cope and make decisions about anything!

I asked, no, I actually demanded bereavement counselling right after Craig's funeral. I knew I needed help. I was scared to be left alone to deal with these intense emotions and thoughts by myself. I attended one incredibly horrible appointment with a psychologist shortly after Craig died. He abruptly ended our session, his parting words to me were 'you are just going to have to get through it.' I raced out to the carpark, ending up in my car, alone and howling my eyes out, feeling worse than when I went in.

It got better. I found it beneficial working with a social worker from the palliative care unit that supported us briefly before Craig passed away. He helped me with strategies and coping skills in the early weeks, but after a couple of months, I felt I needed and wanted more, so I thought about finding a support group I could attend.

My search led me to discover very few options and I was both shocked and disappointed to find that a huge thing like losing your spouse had such limited resources available. I discussed this with my social worker and he agreed there was not much out there. I read books, researched articles, found groups on social media to join, but I found I outgrew some of those quite quickly – some felt like a place to go to dump your emotions. A safe space where you were heard and understood when the rest of the world did not, or could not, bear your pain, however there did not seem to be a way to move forward. I felt stuck and I was looking for more. I was searching for hope. I wanted to know it could get better, that I would feel different and life would be more than this wretched, painful existence where I did not feel connected.

To anything.

I spoke to some people who had attended different support groups in the past, hoping to be directed to something helpful, and I learned their experiences were not all positive. I felt like I was hitting brick walls. I was looking for something to pull me out of my grief, toward healing and overcome the feeling of being trapped in it. The way some described their experience – that it felt like they were pulled into their grief, not out of it, and that was not what I was looking for.

I did stumble across something, on Father's Day 2019. The Grief Recovery Method®. I was instantly intrigued by this and wanted to know more. I contacted the Director of The Grief Recovery Institute, Australasia. From our conversation, I learned that not only could I access a program to help me, I could become certified to help others, too. The training was in March 2020.

When you get used to the feeling of being numb and incapable of experiencing positive emotions, it came as a bit of a shock when, for the first time in months, I felt a tiny flutter of excitement in my belly and I burst into tears. I was feeling flooded with mixed emotions. I honestly never thought I would feel excited about anything again.

I was also relieved.

Relieved that this part of me was not broken, after all. The Grief Recovery Method® was exactly what I was looking for. And I knew then I wanted to provide the very thing I had been searching for, to help other people feeling like me. It became very clear that it was not enough for me to work through my own grief, and leave others like me without any support. I felt a responsibility to change this.

I signed up. I booked flights and accommodation. And then I waited 6 months, not focusing on much else beyond March 2020. It was almost all I could think about.

In the meantime, I was still searching for ways to understand and heal. Grief fascinated me. I was acutely aware of the impact it was having on my entire existence. But also, how incredibly uncomfortable it made people around me, how people avoided me because they did not know how to talk to me.

And just how unprepared and inept we are as a society to deal with grief, that of our own as well as others.

I openly shared my grief experience, on social media, raw, vulnerable and honest. I wanted to let people know I was struggling with this huge derailment in my life. I felt so far away from the person I knew, they knew, and my whole life, sparking some to suggest I should write a book.

Here is one of the posts:

⟡⟡

19 August 2019

Self-care means listening to your body and doing what it needs.

So that is the reason for this.

I have to say it is exhausting being me right now.

I am back at work in a capacity I am comfortable with, but I have to manage my energy. I find I am quite low on energy after classes, so I have to take time out to restore and prepare.

If I retreat quickly, it's just me doing what I need for me.

I am saying yes to more than I was, but not forcing myself to do so.

Some people avoid me, but I also do avoid people. I know I have been someone who was a high-energy and intense individual who can be loud and animated ... not so much at the moment. And that is also something I have to limit my time around.

I am working on things and I am still having bereavement counselling to be able to ... survive losing Craig.

Why am I sharing this?

Because it is who I am now, and I have always believed it is important to be honest and authentic.

It helps me. And my family and friends say it helps them help and support me. And they are doing a fantastic job. I need people around me.

And it's not a sign of weakness to ask for help or to take time out for you.

I know others who are going through a similar time right now, and while our grief is our own, we share similar experiences. It might help people understand us better, while we find our way in our new existence.

When I reached out to other widows about writing a book about grief experiences, I was amazed at how many women came forward. They said they wanted to help me by sharing their experiences as well, in the hope it will help other women and men who have lost their person, their beloved life partner and spouse. They, like me, wanted to help you, dear reader, have the things, the advice and support we wished were available to us.

All of the people who shared their stories with me had a devastating, life-changing, tragic experience when they, like me, lost the love of their life.

While we share the loss of our husband or wife, our circumstances are different.

Our grief is our own.

Each of us had a unique relationship with the person we lost and our feelings are valid, real and intense. It does not matter how our loved ones died. We all miss them.

Every. Single. Day.

When Craig died, I learned from other widows, about 'The Club'. Someone said to me something along the lines of 'you have joined our club' and it was said with empathy, and genuine concern for me. However, I am here to tell you it is the *worst* club on earth, without a doubt. Nobody willingly signs up for a membership to this club because it comes with a very high price.

And we did not have a choice. Although I would rather not be in this club, there is something uniquely unifying about it, an extraordinary connection to others who have loved and known devastating loss.

And survived.

There is wisdom, sadness, empathy, truth, pain, compassion, support and hope here, born only from the unique, harsh and incomparable circumstances which bought us all to this place. We have our own paths and continue to walk them, but in these pages we leave a trail of breadcrumbs for you to follow on your path. It is our hope that what is shared with you, offers some gentle support, kind words that act like a warm hug and knowledge you are not alone. May this be a place to fall into when it feels like the world has stopped listening or caring, to find some sound advice and strategies, comfort and an occasional smile to help you navigate your way through this, your grief.

How to Read This Book

This book is written to show how grief may show up in your life. None of us were prepared for the onslaught that hit us when we lost our respective spouses. The stories and experiences are shared to offer some awareness of what you may feel, in order to let you know that you are not alone, and you are not losing your mind.

If you are looking for diagnostics, you will not find it here. There are no fancy labels and specific details about stages of grief. I have my views about this, and to give you some idea, I feel that these can be counterproductive. By giving you a fancy name, defining it and putting a loose time frame around how long it will last, I personally feel that we give our power over to grief, it defines how we perceive ourselves, pulls us into it rather than out. Grief is hard enough as it is without feeling locked into phases, stages, labels and timeframes. To me, it does not serve any benefit for getting through the day, knowing these things … It still just feels like shit.

Everyone will have a unique relationship with their loss and it will look different in each situation. You may not identify with parts or any of these experiences, and that is ok. However, having been through the ravages of loss and grief, and now helping others to work through and heal from theirs, the aim of my book is to share some strategies and coping mechanisms to help you manage as you meet your grief, get to know it and learn to adjust, navigate and move forward with it in your new existence.

If I can help just one other person who's gone through this, then I feel like writing this book will have been worthwhile.

Jodie x

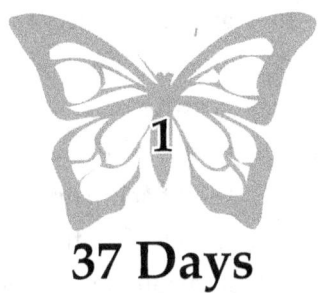

37 Days

'Tis a fearful thing to love what death can touch.
A fearful thing to love, to hope, to dream, to be
– to be,

And oh, to lose.

A thing for fools, this, and a holy thing, a holy thing to love. For your life has lived in me, your laugh once lifted me, your word was gift to me.

To remember this brings painful joy.

'Tis a human thing, love, a holy thing, to love what death has touched.'

~ Yehuda HaLevi ~

We barely had time to get used to the idea Craig was sick before he was gone. Pancreatic cancer does not usually present with symptoms until it is in its advanced stages. It is silent and aggressive.

Like so many other people who are diagnosed with this insidious disease, we learned back pain is a symptom. Craig had complained of a sore back, but this was not unusual at first. At 52, he would occasionally mention his 'back was playing up'. It was not a serious problem, but it occurred on and off over a few years.

He was on his feet a lot at work, and when he set himself a task, he would work hard to get it done. I would catch him playing a vigorous game of tug-of-war with our dog, he would throw himself into odd jobs around the house, help out a mate with moving or a project, or because he loved working out, probably overdo it when exercising. With some massage, physio or chiropractic treatment, it would settle down and he would be back to normal.

Not this time. This time it just did not get better. And we had no reason to suspect cancer was the cause. Why would we?

Another thing, Craig had participated in a male ageing study over a number of years, undergoing different health assessments and tests as part of the study. He was actually preparing for another one just prior to his diagnosis. To our knowledge, he was in good physical health.

But then a couple of other symptoms became present, again, they were not serious or unusual complaints for Craig. However, when you put them together with the back pain, and you search pancreatic cancer symptoms (they told us not to, but I did just this one time). There it was. Like a stinging slap, it hit me!

From the moment we learned of his diagnosis, it seemed we were running on a different program. We were pushing through in survival mode and it was fight or flight all the way. As the days rolled over it became clear we were not going to have as much time as we first anticipated, from the information we were given. I remember saying to my social worker during a counselling session, that it felt like we were in a deadly game of chess, every move we made, cancer had other plans and stopped us in our tracks. Check. Every single time we tried something, there we were with a new 'thing' to face, to overcome. Check. We were running out of time and options. The King was under attack and there was nothing we could do to protect him.

Checkmate.

According to the Pancare Foundation and PanKind, The Australian Pancreatic Cancer Foundation websites, survivor rates have not changed significantly in 40 years. Only 10.7% survive 5 years. Two thirds of patients diagnosed will die within the first year.

A Time to Get Real

This is a time to get really honest and truthful about your situation and ensuring the people in your life who are closest to you understand the gravity of what this diagnosis and prognosis means. It is about making the most of what you have, when you don't have much time.

Your life and your priorities change. Insignificant details fall away. It all becomes so clear. We should be doing this every day – right now – *but if ever there is a time to communicate openly and honestly and be present in every moment, this is it, and that is exactly what we did.* 37 days is not long. We thought we had more time, from what we were advised, but cancer called the shots.

We did not know how long we had, but we made the decision to make the time we had, count. We achieved a lot in this time, my most treasured memory was our wedding. It was important and special for both of us. We planned our wedding, thinking we had months ahead to spend as husband and wife. We had set a date, but we had to bring it forward due to Craig's deteriorating health.

Sadly, he passed away the following day. I was heartbroken.

The other was something that had always been extremely important to Craig, for as long as I have known him. Organ donation. While it might be difficult and uncomfortable, it is the time to have these conversations about *your* situation, wishes, organ donation, and making final arrangements. It was Craig's wish to donate his corneas, and give the gift of sight to someone who is unable to see. Words cannot describe how it feels to be in the position to carry out and honour his wish, knowing that his gift will make such a difference to someone else's life. It means everything to me that together, we were able to make it happen.

A number of widows discussed with me that their significant other was diagnosed with some form of terminal cancer. Their seemingly healthy husbands and wives experienced some health issues or changes and soon after were delivered the devastating news, and their worlds shattered.

It is an extremely unusual, quite indescribable period of time. On one hand the reality of the situation is that you are in the fight for life, the ups, the downs and the really scary and confronting stuff. Yet in the midst of all this, is a very special time of connection. A time when bonds are strengthened, where love and intimacy transcend anything you have ever known about love and intimacy, in a way I find difficult to articulate, and I honestly think it is only through such an experience can it be fully understood, appreciated and regarded. As a lovely man said to me 'we fell in love all over again' describing to me the time spent together during his wife's final months of her illness. And that really resonated with me.

Every situation is different with a terminal diagnosis.

Options may or may not be offered depending on the stage and type of illness.

Time frames will differ and how to proceed will be determined by medical advice, attitudes, opinions and choices.

Some people may choose treatment, others may not. Some may have the option of surgery, others may not.

Regardless of the choices available to you, and what situation you are in, nothing prepares you for the 'shit sandwich' you are served.

Getting up and getting on with the day became difficult, as the uncertainty of our situation and concern for Craig meant everything else paled in significance. He insisted he was fine, and I should go to work. He was not one for a fuss. We were preparing for him to commence treatment, and I just wanted to be with him.

Sometimes the stress and worry would show itself in the most simple everyday things. I tried to keep it together, for him, but sometimes it all got a bit too much. I remember one particular morning, I was preparing my breakfast, putting my cereal in the microwave oven. I was feeling emotional and my stomach was in knots but I was trying to stay in control. The microwave stopped working and my breakfast was still not warm. I swore at it and burst into tears. Craig came into the kitchen and grabbed me in a hug as I continued to cry and berate the microwave into his chest. After a few seconds, he half laughed at me, and said 'it's just a microwave' with a smile, and I said to him 'it's not just the fucking microwave, is it?' and he looked at me, nodded and we hugged while I cried, holding him so tight. When I wiped my tears away and he said 'you ok?' I replied 'yep'. He nodded and said 'so you gonna go to work?' and I answered 'yep' and he said 'good', gave me a squeeze and a smile, watched me grab my cold cereal out of the microwave, then left me to eat my breakfast.

Once Craig's treatment started, things escalated with side-effects and additional health concerns, medications and dietary changes. Things became unpredictable when we had to drop everything and rush to the hospital if he spiked a temperature. Our life was changing so fast and in a very short time, our happy relatively care-free existence was becoming unrecognizable. We felt like we were no longer the drivers of our own destiny, we were mere passengers travelling at high-speed and out of control.

At this point, I have to be candid with you. While I understand you may be interested to learn more about my husband's illness and how we managed this, how he handled everything thrown at him, Craig was quite a private person and wasn't one for attention or fuss. During his short fight with cancer, only family and very close friends knew the full story. Everyone else was told only what we felt they needed to know. We had our reasons.

As I write these early pages, I am extremely mindful of this. I appreciate you may feel the need for me to share more. I get it, he was a great guy, he was popular, he cared about others and he was my rock. I mean, after the doctor had told him he had pancreatic cancer, as we left the surgery, he turned and said to her how sorry he was that it couldn't be a good day at work for her if she is having to deliver that news. Yeah, he did.

But as we had maintained all along, it is not up for discussion, and I remain respectful of his wishes.

What I can tell you about my husband is that he was incredibly brave, pragmatic, selfless in his concern for others, maintained his sense of humour and continued to be the amazing human we knew and loved, until the day he passed away.

Setting Boundaries

From the moment we knew what we were dealing with, we set some very firm boundaries, but it did not feel like boundary setting at the time. It was survival mode and it was about protecting him, me and our family. As I said above, we only told family and close friends the real deal. Everyone else was told what we felt they needed to know. Of course, we had to expect people would be curious as to why I had to cancel many plans and work commitments in order to attend appointments with Craig. Just giving a weak excuse would become tiresome and irritating, so we decided to tell people part of the truth, he was undergoing some treatment for cancer, and I needed to be available to take him to appointments. Enough information meant people were more understanding, no objections and no issues when it came to changing plans.

Inevitably, people asked what type of cancer and what stage, and they were firmly told that was not up for discussion. And like a carefully executed campaign, we stayed on message, putting out only what we wanted to share, knowing if it came back to us via an unexpected random source, it would likely be consistent with what we had expressed.

We knew what we were up against. The last thing we needed was other people coming back to us with their Google horror stories, misinformation or own personal accounts that were not helpful to our situation. We had our own race to run, and we could not allow ourselves to be slammed with distractions and scaremongering. We were in survival mode and this was about self-preservation.

And without being defeatist and fatalistic, it is not helpful, either to engage with 'stay positive, stay strong' or the 'happy, positive, you-hang-in-there, you-can-beat-it cancer talk', with people who do not understand the odds are stacked against you.

Shut it down. Quick.

Boundaries are something you'll no doubt be learning about now or needing to institute very soon. When something like cancer lands in your life people want to know more than they need to, and it requires strength in boundary setting to state the kind of thing I've stated here, and it's important to honour that. You don't need the added pressure of managing others' opinions and judgement of your choices or how you choose to deal with the hand you have been dealt.

The medical team will guide and advise, and of course, the patient will do what they can and take on board what the medical team suggest, participate in trials, anything in the hope to get the upper hand on cancer, reduce symptoms, and buy more time, but the reality is that it does not always work.

Learning About Grief

This book, what this story is about is how, through losing my husband, I came to learn a thing or two about grief – the hard way. As I said, I had no idea what it would feel or look like, or the way it would show up in my life.

For me, losing Craig highlighted a significant lack in our development as a society. We will all experience loss in some way, and yet, we are ill-equipped to deal with it. We simply are not taught what happens to us and how we deal with our feelings when we lose someone we love. Although I am no stranger to loss, I have never experienced the all-consuming, crushing, overwhelming broken-ness that hit me full force when Craig died.

It slammed hard, fast and knocked the wind out of me, turned my life completely upside down. I was not prepared for the onslaught. It broke me, I could not get through a cup of coffee without breaking down in floods of tears. And there seemed to be a permanent lump in my throat whenever I tried to have a conversation. Grief crawled all over me and infiltrated every cell of my being.

But I am not alone. Others who have had the life-changing and devastating loss of a husband, wife or close loved one have also shared aspects of their grief journey, because everyone grieves in their own way, and it is *all valid*. We all learned that some people act weird around you when you are grieving, and I wanted to put a bright spotlight on it. There are similarities in the way grief affects us, and there are differences, too. I want you to see that grief is a unique experience, and in Grief

Recovery®, we explain all grief is experienced at 100 per cent, and we should *absolutely not* compare our losses.

Grief does not show up the same for everybody. Like many other aspects of life, it certainly is not one-size-fits-all. In the beginning it feels like you have very little control over how you feel, act, think, behave and interact with others ... There is no right or wrong way to grieve – you just experience it in your own way, and you feel what you feel, and it is ok to do that.

I was asked specifically by another widow to put this in this book for you.

She told me what she has learned is we need to grieve and grieve well. We need to do more of it. Grieve as much as you can. Grieve this devastating thing that has happened. For the person you lost, all that they were – spouse, partner, all that they did and the connection, intimacy, friendship, companionship. Grieve for your life together, your past and your memories. Grieve for your future you have also lost, the plans, hopes and dreams, the growing old together. Grieve. Allow yourself to feel the feelings that come up.

Some widows chose to be alone while others felt safer to explore feelings knowing there were people around them. Some found journaling helped to get emotions out. A few had counselling, others chose not to. Some went to bereavement groups, others said it was the last place they wanted to go. It is up to you how you choose to explore your feelings, but grieving your loss is important.

Be aware that some of these feelings can be very uncomfortable. Some people do not know how to handle such intense, strong emotions. You may want to ensure you are having some level of therapeutic treatment or support to work through your grief, especially if you are prone to panic attacks, suffering from anxiety or having thoughts of self-harm or suicide.

Jodie's Tips:

You are dealing with some heavy stuff and it is all new and very scary. You are allowed to protect your person, your family and yourself. Setting boundaries will help you manage your situation and focus on what is important.

Boundary setting tips:

- » Discuss what information you are comfortable sharing with people outside your family and support people, and stick to it.

- » Have a response planned for those who are concerned, but also curious and want to know more.

- » Be firm, just say it is not up for discussion. They only need to know what you want them to.

- » Don't allow yourself to be pulled into unhelpful and distracting conversations, just excuse yourself, stay on message or change subject.

- » Understand that grief is as individual as your fingerprint and that you may experience new, weird and foreign emotions.

What We Covered

- A time to get real
- Setting boundaries
- Learning about grief

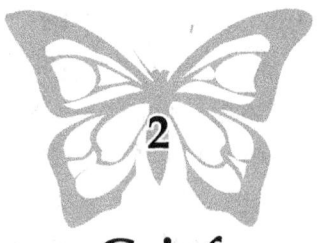

Grief
– The New Companion

'No one ever told me that grief felt so much like fear'

~ C.S Lewis ~

When Craig died, Grief walked in, kicked off its shoes, slumped down in a chair saying 'if you are making a coffee, I'll have one, too' and made itself right at home. And just like any unwelcome house-guest, it was persistent, messy, unpredictable, exhausting and at times, volatile.

Sometimes it was like taking a screaming toddler out in public, except no one else could see and hear it, but it felt like all eyes were on you, anyway.

Grief becomes a constant companion that never leaves you alone. You cannot give it to someone else to hold while you take a break. It is relentless. There are times it quietly rests, like the calm before the storm, lulling you into a false sense of security.

In these times you may feel like you are in a foggy haze – and it has a name … 'widow-brain', yes, it is a thing – and you lose yourself, your ability to function, and time, don't ask me how, you just … disconnect and it happens in this fog.

A lot of widows talk about experiencing widow-brain. You feel like your brain has turned to mush, you cannot concentrate, you forget things, people tell you things and you can't – and don't – really hear them, and it just feels hazy.

Roller Coaster of Grief Emotions

Then without warning, Grief can erupt with ferocious energy, unleashing an explosive cocktail of emotions leaving you feeling anxious, vulnerable and fragile, overwhelming your ability to focus, make decisions and just string a sentence together.

And *those* panic attacks are the worst. A tidal wave of panic hit me from out of nowhere. It literally felt like it engulfed me. My heart pounded in my chest, and I felt like I couldn't breathe properly. My stomach was in knots. It felt like something was crawling all over me, restricting me. I just started pacing up and down, to try and shake it off, crying and feeling overwhelmed with fear. In these moments, I actually feared I would not get through this. I have never felt so incredibly helpless and unsure of how to cope with the depths these panic attacks took me to. I am not exaggerating. I told my mum I could not – was not going to live the rest of my life doing this, if this kept happening. Because it was horrendous. I do remember her looking at me wide-eyed – I can only imagine how concerning it would be to see your daughter so distraught and in such a dark place. But she just spoke to me in a quiet, calming voice, and did not appear to show any sign of panic herself.

To say I was scared is an understatement. Feeling like there was no way to overcome this was petrifying. My previous losses, my 'grief experiences', while I remember feeling sadness, lost, and the significant people – grandparents, family, friends, acquaintances and other people who were important to me, who I admired and respected, and dearly missed – did not feel like this and did not 'prepare' me for losing Craig. I did not know grief could or would feel like fear and anxiety. I did not know grief would come crashing into my life, create explosions of intense emotions I could not control or understand, and it was as though it occupied every aspect of my life … waiting to prey on me when I least expected it.

This made me feel like I was losing my mind and behave in ways that made no sense. I cannot recall ever having any experience like it, and I had days where I thought I would just end it if it did not go away.

One day I decided to confront the panic attack head on. I had used a technique with clients regarding food cravings, when the urge to disappear into the ice cream bucket seemed the only way to deal with certain emotions. Instead, sit with the emotions mindfully and explore what your body is trying to tell you, what do you really feel?

So I decided I would do this with the panic attack. I felt it hit and my first instinct was to start pacing and let it suck the air from my lungs like it usually did. But I decided to look it in the eye and say, 'Ok, come on then. Let's do this' and I sat and let it completely engulf me. I remember feeling my heart race, and I breathed deeply in and out, I mindfully took note of how it felt like something was sitting on me, my eyes were closed and as I let it unleash, I just focused on my breathing. It was scary, I cried the whole time and I remember saying 'no' over and over as if it would listen to me. Like a wave it gradually built in intensity to the point where I almost gave in to pacing and screaming. It was like it rose to the challenge, it felt like something was pinning me down but grabbing at me and shaking me at the same time. It felt like it was determined to beat me. But I sat and continued to breathe, noticing I was trembling and my whole body was tense.

Then suddenly, I was aware that it was easing off, slowly. I kept breathing and opened my eyes not sure what I expected to see, but I focused on my surroundings, mindfully looking at my chair, the picture of my dog, the tv. It eased off and I started to feel like I had won. I had shown it I was in control. I cried hard and loud.

The next time the panic reared its head, I started breathing and mindfully sat into it. It was not as intense and it did not last as long. And the time after that, less again. Eventually I noticed I wasn't having these horrendous attacks at all.

Other widows also said they had no warning. When I talk about this now, I hear people say, they either know from experiencing it or know someone who has. So how is it that we still find out about it the hard way – having it show up in our lives with no warning and no plan to cope with it? This is the stuff we should be discussing and bringing some awareness to. It sucks to find out this way.

A few of us expressed a real sense of being disconnected from life. Everything feels so insignificant and unimportant. It is so hard to be interested in anything when you feel removed from the life you knew and have the realisation that you no longer feel a sense of purpose. I felt like I was on a treadmill

– it was moving but I was not going anywhere. I honestly felt like life had little meaning to it.

Others felt angry.

Angry at God.

Angry at the situation they found themselves in.

Angry for having their person ripped from their life.

Angry at their husband for leaving them to carry on with life without them.

Angry because they were not meant to die so young, and there was no reason why they should have died. It just didn't make sense that someone could die when there was every reason to survive … there was early CPR and paramedics and medical intervention … but still, sadly and tragically, they did die.

Numbness is another common experience, and this can vary in duration. Some described feeling this way for almost a year, and just getting out of bed is the big achievement for the day. Some women said they shut down, put up a wall and showed little emotion.

Like me, many of the women felt anxious and fragile. We felt anxious about getting anxious around people or in public places.

Some said they felt like they were in shock for a really long time. And others felt 'complete and utter heartbreak', despair and hopelessness.

Dark Humour

Then, the use of dark humour, or as some call it, 'widow-humour'. You start making jokes about yourself for being foggy and scatterbrained, or about things that unexpectedly amuse you, observations of your new existence or the way some people can be weird around you. You may even use it to describe aspects of the loss you have experienced. Others are not sure how to respond, they look awkwardly around to see if others find it funny, and you can see them thinking, 'should I laugh?'. You can see them trying to work out what is an appropriate way to respond, which in itself, can be amusing, too.

You may find you get really honest. You say how you feel, what you think, as one widow said, 'call out people on their bullshit'.

She became so blunt. She described a situation where she was having a conversation with someone and they were really uncomfortable about grief and death. She asked them 'why are you so uncomfortable? This happened to me!'

She said 'I am not going to sugar coat it, I am not Willy Wonka, you know. I can't be in charge of your uncomfortableness and mine!'.

One thing is for sure, it is unpredictable, and you can be brought to tears by the most unlikely thing. You will feel different hour by hour, not just day by day. I borrowed that famous line from *Forrest Gump,* the scene where he is sitting on the park bench talking about life being like a box of chocolates. I would tell people I was like the box of chocolates, cos they'd just never know what they were going to get if they spent any time with me.

Grief absolutely turns your life into a roller coaster of highs and lows. The first time I asked my friends to come visit me after Craig's funeral, I sent a message saying, 'be sure to buckle your seatbelt for the roller coaster you are about to ride'. To which one of my friends responded. 'hey, I love roller coasters! Count me in!'.

And to me, that was just simply the best response. Knowing my friends could be comfortably uncomfortable hanging out with me and my grief, accepting that whatever was going to happen would happen and we would just deal with it.

Together.

All of these emotions and feelings happen on their own, or alongside other emotions simultaneously. Part of the feeling that you are losing your mind is that you are bouncing around from one to another in the space of seconds and you have no control. And just when you think you have regained some composure you are off on the roller coaster again.

Identity and Loss of Identity

Prior to this sudden and disastrous upheaval to our lives, this is not who I was. This was not my reality.

I knew who I was, and I now realise more than ever, that I liked that version of me.

And I really miss her. A lot.

I knew my place in the world and I was a confident, independent, positive, fun, animated and outgoing, energetic woman who was always open to a challenge, even the scary ones, and I was happy. I was part of a couple, living life on our terms and had a future of hopes and dreams ahead of us.

Cancer and grief took that away from me.

I did not know who I was anymore. I just did not recognise my life anymore. 37 days is all it took to completely undermine everything I knew and felt about myself. I did not identify with being vulnerable and fragile, yet here I was cloaked in it from head to toe. My head was a mess. I had trouble making decisions. I did not feel connected to anything. I barely knew what day it was. It is alarming, distressing and just plain scary to find yourself questioning your own identity, literally asking yourself, 'who am I now?' and not having any answers.

Not only had I lost the person I was supposed to grow old with, my best friend, life partner and husband, I had lost myself.

Other widows I spoke with said they had a similar experience. One lady described how she felt like she had not only lost her sense of identity, she lost her confidence in the simplest of tasks. Even driving her car, she broke out in a sweat and she says it was like she 'just forgot how to'. She describes having to make phone calls and tend to the business of notifying people and organisations of her husband's passing, and how it felt like she just 'did not know how to go about it'.

Again, this is a woman who has a career, identified as an independent, strong, confident and empowered woman prior to this, and is suddenly overwhelmed and having panic attacks, has no confidence in her ability to do the basic things, things that she considered simple everyday tasks. The impact of grief undermined her mental capacity. When this happens, it is extremely overwhelming and scary.

She also spoke of how her memory let her down, she forgot her own phone number and had to take notes on everything as she could not retain information.

Another lady said 'I had lost my sense of identity – I was part of a couple. It was always "we not me" and "us not I". I didn't know how to function unless I was part of a couple'.

You feel like part of you is missing. And waking up in the morning in those first early days after your person dies, there is that confused daze, where the reality has not kicked in, you think, 'I have to get up, go to the hospital, I have to go see him, oh wait, hang on, no, he isn't there, he has gone', and then there is that ache, deep in your chest, the sinking feeling in your gut as you become aware, again, of your reality. For those first early days, you experience that loss over and over again and again, like it is that day, on repeat.

Adjusting to a New Normal

It takes time to get used to this new period of your life. It is not a race and again, there are no rules.

You will find you are adjusting. Adapting. Navigating. Learning. Trialling.

Make sure you do ask for help with things you find hard or just can't do, whether it is internet issues, leaky taps or gardening. Get the support you need from family, friends, or pay someone to take care of the gutters that need cleaning or gates that need fixing.

Please understand you don't have to have or know the answers to the questions:

'What are you going to do now?'
'How will you manage?'
'Are you financially ok?'
'Will you stay in your house or will you move?'
'Are you going/when will you go back to work?'
'What do you want?'

Again, having some boundaries around what you will discuss, and with whom, will help you manage these. Or delegate someone to step in and take care of the talk, the questions and the people you can't deal with.

You need to allow yourself to grieve and these answers will come to you in their own time. Saying that, time frames will vary for each person, depending on their situation.

Doing what is right for you is what is important. Don't be rushed by others thinking they know what is best for you if you don't feel it is in your best interests.

Some women returned to work after only a few days or weeks thinking routine would be good, to focus on something else. Some said that in hindsight, that was probably not a great decision, and should have taken more time off. Others found they felt judged because they were attending meetings or back at work. Some people were telling them it was too soon, while other co-workers had assumed that they were ok, if they were back at work, business as usual. However, when a widow did have days where they struggled and got upset, they did not feel like people understood they were still grieving during this time and actually were not ok.

Some days you will feel like you are having a good day, and things will go smoothly. Other times, it is an all-consuming effort from the minute you drag yourself out of bed, force yourself to get dressed, maybe eat something and constantly tell yourself, 'come on, you will be ok once you get there'. Sometimes you believe it, other days it is quickly followed up with 'who am I kidding?'

The whole day is one giant self-pep-talk. Many of us experienced some difficulty returning to the workplace. The thought of going back to work with grief on board creating havoc with your cognitive processes and feeling like your emotions are all competing to be let out at the same time, is stressful and makes you doubt your ability to cope. You are already in fight, flight or freeze mode, and it is absolutely debilitating. And then there are the people you work with, some not sure what to say to you, others avoid you like the plague and those who don't think before speaking and 'word salads' fall out of their mouths. We all had an experience we could recall, and some were so very similar.

One widow describes the time someone at the office greeted her first thing in the morning with 'oh you don't seem to be your usual cheerful self today, are you having a bad day?' She said this person sat down on a chair and started to talk about how they deal with a bad day. She said she explained this is more than just a bad day. 'My husband died'. She blurted 'this is how my life looks now, this is me getting used to my new life'. Then, after explaining to this person how much of an effort it is to just get up in the morning, and honestly, how it would be so much easier to not come in to work at all, she finished with 'so, sorry I am not jumping around for joy, but isn't it enough that I am here? What, I have to perform for you as well?'.

Change

As you start to navigate your new normal, other people, while still there for you, will go on with their lives. You might find yourself thinking, 'how can everyone be so normal and act like nothing has changed while I am over here, barely holding together, my whole world has changed and I am trying to deal with the gaping hole in my life!'

Everything has changed.

It feels so lonely. It is hard. We had no choice. We did not ask for this. And most widows I spoke with appreciated someone just calling it out for what it was, no holding back. I heard it a few times … 'It is just shit'.

A significant person in your life dies. All aspects of your life change.

This is one of the biggest learning curves that we discovered. And this is something not everyone is aware of as they go back to their lives, as time rolls on. For some who attend a funeral, they may find some closure. They say their goodbye.

For many widows and widowers, this is not the case. In the weeks and months after, is where it can be incredibly confronting and difficult.

Everything changes. *Everything!*

- The way you do your grocery shopping.
- The way you eat. So many widows describe the difficulty and the lack of interest in cooking for one.
- The way you sleep. Some widows found comfort sleeping on their husband's side of the bed. Others would sit up late and put off going to bed. Some could not sleep in their own bed.
- The way you do laundry.
- The way you think. Your perception of things changes, you see things through a different lens.
- Your tolerance changes. Some widows say they can no longer tolerate small talk and have a very powerful 'bullshit radar'.
- For some, you are suddenly alone, having to parent your children.
- The jobs around the house that were allocated 'his job' and 'my job', well, they all become your job.
- Your morning routine.

- Your evening routine.
- The way you pay your bills.
- Even watching television, shows you used to watch together are just not the same anymore.

It *all* changes.

And as the weeks turn into months, and months turn into a year, and so on, people around you do not understand how all of this change is a big period of adjustment and the impact it has on you. Your life was full of them – they were everywhere. You did so many things together. You discussed everything. You made a lot of decisions together. You always 'checked in' out of consideration when plans were made. You worked as a team to manage the household and kids. They were the one you looked forward to a quiet Saturday night with, just being at home … together.

And then they are gone.

And their absence is present in everything you do.

People don't live it so they don't see it.

Unless you tell them, they don't know it.

And even then, they don't understand it.

Unless you have lived it, you just don't really comprehend what this feels like.

So be gentle with yourself. Acknowledge things. Express how you feel about these changes.

Structure and Routines

In the weeks and months after Craig's death, I decided I needed the structure of some new routines. Everything was different now and it wasn't 'we' but 'me' running the household.

I got in touch with a guy I went to school with who has his own landscaping/gardening business. I asked him to help me with maintaining my garden and cleaning gutters etc. I struggle with this stuff at the best of times, and it was stressful seeing what needed to be done and feeling overwhelmed by it all. It took the pressure off me feeling like I had to do it all.

One of my lovely friends gifted me a delivery box of meals to try out. I had been struggling with meal preparation as I could not muster motivation to cook for myself, and I realised I needed to change that. My first box arrived – I loved it, and I continued to order these meals for several months. Not only was it the convenience of it being delivered to my house, but I was cooking proper meals from scratch. I started to get excited about ordering my meals, learning some great new recipes and it was nice to experience the aromas in my kitchen again, cooking with fresh herbs, trying new ingredients and making my own dressings.

Getting back to exercise was more appealing when I walked with other people. I would say yes if I was invited or I would ask others to join me. It felt less like a chore and I appreciated the company, too.

My friend asked me to join her gym, saying she would appreciate having a training partner for extra motivation and accountability, going 2-3 times a week with her. Once I had been a few times, I started going most mornings during the week, even the days my friend was unavailable to go. I did not join any classes and just did what I felt comfortable doing. I did not put pressure on myself to work hard, just committed to doing 45-60 mins of resistance training and added some light cardio. Not being an early riser previously, I found myself wondering how I became this 5:30am morning person going to the gym every week day, but it felt right, I was enjoying it and I just did it.

Then COVID-19 shut us down.

I did not return to the gym.

Your grief has shown up and it feels like you have a new companion constantly demanding your attention. Life as you knew it has changed and so has your ability to function. You are bouncing around from one emotion to the next, your body and your mind seem to no longer belong to you, you have no control over what is happening. One minute you feel like you are walking around in a haze, and the next, you are in the trenches fighting it out with anxiety and panic.

Every single aspect of your life has changed, from the moment you open your eyes in the morning, and you feel like only you really understand the gravity of this as you go about your day.

The empty space.

The unwanted solitude.

The undeniable absence.

The constant ache.

The deafening roar of silence.

Jodie's Tips:

The loss of your person changes everything. Grief impacts your ability to cope with these changes, as your emotions bounce all over the place. Because your emotions are so volatile, and your decision-making capabilities are impaired, holding off on big decisions, if you don't need to make them immediately, is probably a good idea.

Your memory can be unreliable, so making big decisions when you are not thinking clearly could cost you dearly, financially and emotionally.

- » Find people who can help you manage different areas of your life. Help maintaining the garden or cleaning your home, food preparation, a walking or exercise buddy, to either help keep you accountable or for company.

- » When the roller coaster of emotions come, it's time to just go with it. You can be laughing and then crying within minutes, sometimes seconds. You feel so fatigued, and like you have no emotional stability. Just accept this is your grief and express it.

» When you feel like you have lost your sense of identity, it is scary. I found reading books and articles and watching relevant presentations (check out my resources for links) helped me feel 'normal', that what I was experiencing was not uncommon. Understanding these things can happen takes some intensity out of the confusion and anxiety that comes with these foreign emotions. If you can accept this is part of the grieving process then it makes it a little easier to manage.

» If you have to make decisions, talk to someone who is able to help you. Get advice from a trusted financial advisor for managing your finances. Your family and trusted friends might be able to help you problem-solve other decisions you have to make regarding property, family arrangements and returning to work.

» Give yourself time to grieve. Cry, journal, remember there is no right or wrong way, just your way. Feel your feelings.

» Take the pressure off yourself to have all the answers and just be kind to yourself as you navigate this horrid new challenging time.

What We Covered

- The roller coaster of emotions
- Dark humour
- Identity and loss of identity
- Adjusting to a new normal
- Change
- Structure and routines

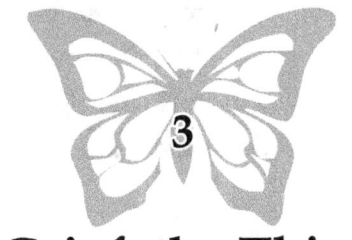

Grief, the Thief

'There is a sacredness in tears. They are not the mark of weakness, but of power. They speak more eloquently than ten thousand tongues. They are the messengers of overwhelming grief, of deep contrition, and of unspeakable love'.

~ Washington Irving ~

Grief has well and truly become your new companion, and it impacts every area of your life. Every pillar and every foundation you've built will be touched. Grief will rob you of your routine, your habits, your health, showing up in places you never realised it could reach.

The Impact on the Body

Not only does Grief completely turn you inside out emotionally and mentally, it takes its toll on you, physically. It is exhausting just being you. Grief is big. It is a powerful, all-consuming beast. It wreaks havoc on your body, robbing you of energy, sleep and concentration. It steals your emotional resilience. It makes you feel unsafe. It completely messes with your appetite. You are in the trenches, and your body is under attack.

Now I get that you may not feel like or even care about anything else other than how lost you feel right now, and you can always revisit this chapter when you feel more interested. However, this part could help you to understand why it may feel like your body is fighting you, too.

This book is about supporting you through your loss and all of the things that I and other widows thought you might find helpful. If you are like me, you are constantly wondering what the hell is wrong with you, and this might explain a few things, and provide you with a sense of how grief is impacting your health.

Grief hangs around and it drains you. It makes you feel tired, low in energy and destroys your motivation. All the information I read said self-care is really important. It is recommended you get enough sleep, exercise and eat well.

Pfft! Yeah right!

Anyone who knows me would expect me to be the first to agree. Under normal circumstances. But I was emotional. I was exhausted. I missed my husband so much I ached, like part of me was missing. I did not care one bit. I was so far removed from life as I knew it. Everything was different. I was different. The last thing I felt like doing was swinging 'round a set of dumbbells, the thought of it was mentally and physically draining.

During the early weeks after Craig died, I would *actually drive* my dog to the dog park and let him run around – at least I was out of the house, getting some fresh air and moving around a little bit. The dog park became my 'happy place'. No one expected anything from me. I could keep to myself, or engage with others if I felt up to it, there were always other dogs there and they would come up for a pat. It gave me a sense of calm. I could just … be.

Walking on the beach is something I have always enjoyed doing and found washes away any stress or internal dialogue, so I did that at times, too.

It is important to find a space or activity that helps you regain some of that energy. One lady said she found swimming laps in a pool calming, she even called it 'Swim Therapy'. She said she would swim for an hour every morning, it was 'energising and relaxing, and the only thing that helped me not be so anxious and depressed'. She also described how a few months later, she joined a salsa group, taking steps to rebuild her social life.

She said the appeal was the happy music and so many different kinds of people.

She said it saved her life.

Others found writing was therapeutic. One widow in the US said that she would recommend people look at 'Refuge In Grief' and take Megan Divine's writing class. She wrote a blog and then friends encouraged her to write a book. So she did! Her book is about her grief journey called 'Carry On Castle'. It is available on Amazon.

Here are some ways you might find grief is showing up and impacting your body without you realising it: (several were mentioned in Chapter 2)

- A feeling of your stomach in knots
- Feeling exhausted all the time, even when you've slept
- Feeling clumsy
- Feeling shaky or like you have nervousness and tension

- Tightness in the chest, the feeling of a weight on your chest, or chest pains (there is a condition called takotsubo cardiomyopathy otherwise known as 'broken heart syndrome', and symptoms can present similar to those of a heart attack. You should seek medical treatment if you experience this).
- Stomach, gut or digestive issues
- Not sleeping

Changes in appetite is another big one. Some widows said they only ate because someone literally put food in front of them. Most were grateful that someone had cooked some meals to put in the fridge to heat and eat, they didn't have to think about preparing food.

Some of us ate our feelings, giving in to cravings of sweets or savouries. When we crave certain foods (some might call it comfort or emotional eating) the body is looking to soothe or calm itself. It might feel good in the moment, but it does not last.

Your grief can have a huge impact on your immune system, increasing the risk of illness and infections. Grief is a form of stress and when your body is in a state of stress, it is flooded with stress hormones. (Adrenalin, Cortisol and Norepinephrine).

I had some knowledge of how stress impacts your metabolism, ability to lose and maintain weight, and sleep quality from my health and fitness courses. The over production of these hormones puts an enormous strain on the adrenal glands, putting you at risk of adrenal fatigue and increases your chances of chronic illness, weight gain, and other serious conditions.

When I started to increase the intensity of my exercise, I got anxious and just burst into tears. This was a new thing and it felt weird. I did not understand what was happening to me at first … my 'widow-brain' was in full force, I was vague and not as switched on as normal. It was bought to my attention that I was adding stress to an already stressed body, and I was probably in overload.

Light bulb moment! It all came back to me, but it took this chat for me to realise, and make sense to me. I did some of my own research and paid a visit to my GP.

My GP took a blood test and I learned I had a couple of deficiencies, so she recommended supplements. She also reinforced that, under the circumstances, I was 'doing well' and what I was feeling and how my body was responding was quite normal given what I had experienced. I remember saying to her that I felt like I was barely holding on some days, and if this is doing well, I would hate to see what not coping looked like.

If you notice a few body aches and pains, this could also be due to the high amounts of stress hormones surging around your body. The longer the body is under this amount of stress, the greater the risk you are of developing a more serious health concern like chronic illness, heart disease and high blood pressure. It wouldn't hurt to check in with your GP, if you are experiencing any of these issues or if you are concerned. They may also arrange some blood tests to check you out.

Impact on Sleep and Rest

As for sleep, sometimes I did, mostly, I didn't get enough. I would put off going to bed, staying up watching tv or scrolling social media to distract myself. Once I laid my head on the pillow, while the house was quiet and still, my head was making too much noise. A mind no longer distracted, and a big empty bed, of course all I could think about was the circumstances that led to me being in that moment and I would feel all the painful emotions. I would lay there and mostly cry my heart out and I must have cried myself to sleep many times. Sometimes I would just toss and turn watching the hours roll over. I would drift off at some point.

Then morning would come and getting up was the last thing I wanted to do. Other women said the same. I live alone now and had it not been for my dog and 2 cats, I probably would not have put my feet on the floor. But the cats would demand to be fed, meowing at me loudly in the increasingly impatient way that they do, and at some point, my dog would need to go outside to do his business.

So I got up.

Some widows I spoke with had families – they were young pregnant mums, had babies, small children or teenagers – their husbands had been young men, a couple were only in their 30's and 40's. The children still needed their mum to get up and get breakfast, pack lunches and take them to school, to do homework, manage some sort of routine and run them to their sports or excursions and on top of that, deal with the way their children's grief was being expressed – temper tantrums, meltdowns, some noticed their children had become scared and fragile, others had kids asking constant questions, or a child refusing to speak about their dad at all.

For them, staying in bed was not an option.

To be honest, I still don't sleep as well as I used to. I felt I was just settling into a good routine, going to bed around 10pm and getting up at 5:30am to go to the gym. COVID-19 hit and with restrictions, like so many other people across the globe, I could not go about my daily routine and run my business. I did find myself falling back into that late-night procrastination again. What helps me to sleep now, especially in winter, is a warmed-up bed, a cup of calming tea, (a night-time blend that promotes sleep) and reading a few pages of a book in bed.

Impact on the Mind

We talked about poor concentration before, but something worth mentioning here is driving ability. Be careful when you have grief as a passenger in the car with you. The reduced concentration and fogginess of your brain can affect the cognitive processes required for the decisions we make behind the wheel. I had a number of experiences where I found myself thinking, 'jeez, what is wrong with you?', I was making silly errors, late decisions and like everything else, feeling I was on auto pilot.

So I cannot stress enough – *be careful* behind the wheel.

On one occasion I drove into the city to collect a book I had ordered. I wanted to turn right into a side street, so I drove into what I thought was the appropriate lane. I discovered I had actually entered the tram lane! A couple of other drivers honked horns at me but I had nowhere to go, it was a red light and traffic was flowing on the other side of the road. You can imagine the panic as I frantically checked my rear-view mirror and looked ahead to check for approaching trams! Luckily, it was all clear, I just had to wait for the green light, and turn quickly ahead of the guy in the lane next to me, the lane I should have been in, also wanting to turn right. My heart was racing and I was incredibly self-conscious as he kept pointing and mouthing 'tram' at me and all I could do was shrug my shoulders and mouth back 'I know!'

I have to say that when this happened, I was a bit relieved I had spent about 3 hours standing on my driveway peeling and rubbing and wiping my business branding stickers and adhesive off my car! (Distraction level: Expert).

A few days after Craig's funeral I decided, in my foggy and anxious state, the branding had to go. Why? I had changed my surname when we got married, and it had my previous surname. And as I was experiencing so much anxiety when I went anywhere, I didn't want to drive around advertising my whereabouts or my business. I just wanted to be invisible and uncontactable.

Talking to other widows there are many, many ways grief impacts our minds. Here is a list of how these things can show up on day to day basis:

- Widow-Brain
- Difficulty multi-tasking
- Mind fog when driving and following signs
- Difficulty taking in lots of information
- Increase in anxiety when feeling pressure to make a quick decision
- Loss of concentration while reading or watching a movie
- Feeling like you're going to lose it
- Feeling overwhelmed
- Operating on 'auto pilot'
- Reliving the experience of seeing their husband/wife for the last time
- Replaying the traumatic or painful experience in their mind, unable to 'change the channel'
- Feeling the need to keep busy/distracted
- Rash decisions or impaired judgement when making decisions

There are physical signs of grief that show up in our bodies, it is not all emotional. Don't give yourself a hard time for not sticking to your usual eating plan or exercise routine. You do what you have to do to manage the intensity and waves of emotion. You are not going mad. Give yourself permission to grieve and do it your way. The biggest thing I have learned while writing this book is that other people appreciate this conversation because our behaviour, thoughts and actions are 'normalised' by sharing our experiences. It is such a relief when someone writes or speaks about the things you are feeling and experiencing. When I saw that other people had the same or similar experiences, I felt so reassured that what was happening was my grief showing up.

In all its glory.

Be sure to see your GP if you have health concerns or find someone to help you work through your grief, if you feel you need it. There is absolutely no shame in asking for help.

This thing, your grief, is relentless.

It is ok to not be ok, you are not 'doing it (grieving) wrong or right'.

You are doing it your way.

And *that* is ok.

Jodie's Tips:

How to Manage the Impact on the Body:

» Do what feels right for you in the moment. Want to sleep, then sleep. Feel like going for a walk, do that. Feel like watching a movie, that is ok, too. Your body is dealing with a lot. Just don't expect too much from yourself right now. It is ok to do whatever it is that gives you some calm or quiet, what gives it a break from the surges of anxiety, racing thoughts and panic. Self-care may be taking a soak in the bath, a nap or spending some time cuddling your pooch while watching a movie.

» To ensure you are eating, maybe ask family or friends to make your favourite foods or a pot of soup so you can just heat and eat and you are not just defaulting to takeaways, a bag of chips or crackers, wine and cheese for meals. It can happen some days, but you don't want to end up doing it all the time.

It might also be a time you lean on alcohol a little more than usual, too. It is an escape, a distraction. I totally get it. But waking up the next day with a hangover may exacerbate your anxiety or make you feel even more sluggish and low, too. No one could tell me what I should or shouldn't be doing, I was hurting, and had little regard for 'the should's' and I am certainly not going to lecture you. But just something to be aware of, perpetuating a vicious circle of the high from distraction and escape followed by the crashing lows, pulling you back into your heartbroken reality, the ache, the pain and the helplessness. It is just awful. It is not a great place to fall.

How to Have a Better Night's Sleep and Rest:

- If you are having trouble sleeping, there are some good meditation, sleep or mindfulness apps that can be useful to help you relax.
- Maybe some sleep music is more your thing.
- Reading in bed might help you feel drowsy.
- A nice hot shower or soak in the bath before bed can relax tight muscles and ease tension in your body.

- » Try some calming teas. The most well-known for helping sleep quality is Chamomile, either on its own or blended with other herbs. Some blends may suggest adding warm milk as well.

- » Making sure you are comfortable. Some people like a fan on, all year round, the gentle noise and the breeze is what they need to fall asleep. I struggle to get a good sleep if I get cold. Do you need an extra blanket? Use a heatpack or invest in an electric blanket to warm up your bed.

- » Some of us found comfort in sleeping with or wearing an item of clothing that belonged to our husband like a t-shirt or sleeping on his pillow. Some sprayed a little of their husband's aftershave on the clothing or pillow, as well, to offer comfort.

- » Maybe you want to let your pet sleep in your room or on your bed, too. I did. Remember, there are no rules. And no one gets to tell you what to do to look after yourself during this time.

- » If you are concerned that not sleeping is becoming a real problem, speak to your GP.

- » I hope you find something useful here. These are just suggestions to help you work out how you can do what feels right for you.

How to Support Your Mind/Brain:

» A lot of us just want to be heard, have our pain and grief witnessed. Talking about our loss is important. It is part of the grieving process, to help communicate our thoughts and feelings. Being able to talk about our loved ones and our grief can make a griever feel lighter. It can also be quite draining, but I repeat, it is incredibly important.

» NOTE: You need to be able to talk about whatever you want to talk about with someone who will JUST LISTEN. We are going to cover this in more detail in chapter 5.

» Be careful when you are on the road, maybe let others drive where it is appropriate and if travelling long distances, take those rest breaks.

- » Have someone help you make phone calls, send emails and collate information you need for funeral arrangements, probate, insurance, superannuation, banking, tax etc. It can be incredibly overwhelming, emotionally taxing and stressful to deal with the cold, business side of loss. It can be tough to have these hard conversations over and over, and it is emotionally and mentally draining. Outsource that to people where possible. Get them to do as much as they can, and you step in where you have to.

- » And do things in chunks. Just tackle small tasks and don't try to take on too much on your own, especially if you are having a tough day. If you are emotional and feeling overwhelmed, ask yourself, 'can I do it tomorrow?'. Deal with it when you feel like you can cope with it.

- » Buy yourself some time if you feel overwhelmed. Excuse yourself to make a 'phone call' or go to the bathroom. Then, just go find a spot and BREATHE.

What We Covered

- Impact on body
- Impact on sleep and rest
- Impact on the mind

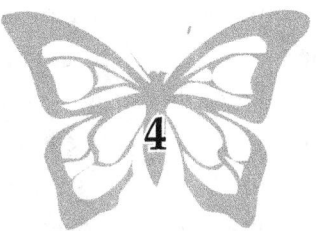

When Grief Just Takes Over

'Grief. The pain now is part of the happiness then. That's the deal'

~ C.S. Lewis ~

Grief goes with you everywhere. You can't just say 'I am popping out, be back in half an hour'. You can't ask someone to hang on to it for little while. It is yours and yours alone. It tags along, throwing a tantrum and kicking, screaming and causing havoc, just like it does at home, except it feels more intense. Your heart races the whole time. I found myself silently repeating over and over, 'please don't let me bump into anyone I know'. Your stomach is in knots and you are on alert. You get back to the car and you stop, close your eyes and breathe. Thank God that is over. And you go home, exhausted, physically drained.

When Getting Anxious about Getting Anxious Becomes Out of Control

I remember the first time I suddenly felt anxious in public. After Craig's funeral, I decided it would be a 'good idea' for our family to go out for dinner rather than have everyone come back to our house, with around 30 people including my family, Craig's family and a couple of our close friends, it seemed sensible. I did not feel I could cope with a lot of people in my home.

I had stopped eating and was sitting, quietly looking around the room at all the people who were there. I watched as they engaged in conversation, eating and drinking, and the thought suddenly occurred to me that under different circumstances, it was highly unlikely that many of these people would ever have met, let alone be in the same room, largely due to geographical location. They were all here because of Craig. And then out of the blue, a wave of panic, and my heart raced, as my inner voice said 'but Craig isn't here'. Suddenly in a room full of people I knew and loved, I felt so alone, and it was overwhelming. The intensity was unbelievable. It completely freaked me out. I asked my friends to take me home – I had to get out of there!

And then it kept happening, and the intensity worsened.

I had to go into the city to drop off some paperwork, soon after Craig's funeral. Of all the places, I bumped into one of my clients in the queue at a government office. At first, I did not see her. She approached me. I looked at her, I had a vague feeling I knew her, but I could not work out how. She spoke to me, I panicked. I fell apart right in front of her. And I felt like I was losing it yet aware enough to feel completely confused and overwhelmed by my reaction, at the same time.

She was served before me. I regained some composure. I approached her and apologised for losing it. She was so lovely. I explained that I did not do public places very well and I wasn't ready to see people. She was so understanding.

Another time I was grocery shopping and as I was putting diced tomatoes in my trolley, the music playing on their sound system set me off. I will never forget this. It was the song 'Sara' by Jefferson Starship. Not a song I have a deep connection to, but on this day, as it played, I was a mess. Tears rolled uncontrollably down my cheeks the whole time I was in the supermarket. I felt exposed. I felt like people could see right through me, that by looking at me they knew – something about me screamed 'my husband just died'.

So then, any time I had to prepare to go out, the thought of leaving the house to do anything became an ordeal. Dealing with legalities, the bank, having to front up with documents whenever I was requested to provide something was so emotionally challenging, stressful, uncomfortable and made me feel weary.

If I went to the shop, I would wear a hat pulled down low, dart in, grab what I needed and get out, eyes down, no looking around for fear of locking eyes with someone I knew … and the thought of that terrified me. Now normally, I would be the type to see someone I knew and wave or go up and say hello, so where the hell did this come from?

The longer I was gone, the more anxious I would become, and it would start to feel like panic. I would feel tears rolling down my cheeks. If I saw someone I knew, I turned and walked the other way, heart racing and breathing fast, feeling like I was about to explode. I did not trust myself to speak to them. I had no idea of what I would do, but it felt like I would just fall apart in front of them. I felt like it was getting worse as time went on and I was beginning to think this was who I was now and how on earth would I be able to go back to work, standing in front of a fitness class with this going on? My life, already in shreds. Now it felt like I was unravelling.

I am not alone. Other widows said they had similar

experiences, and completely understood the getting anxious about getting anxious.

Many have shared experiences where they felt so overwhelmed with anxiety, they had real difficulty leaving the house, so if you are experiencing this, it appears to be quite a common emotional response. You are not alone, and you are not going mad.

Some of us experienced the 'wave'. One minute you are talking to someone and suddenly out of nowhere, a wave of emotion hits and your voice shakes, you feel a lump in your throat, your eyes tingle and tears well up. Sometimes it feels like a tidal wave, at other times just a gentle ebb and flow. It is gone as quickly as it came.

Some had panic attacks like me, but one lady described how she went to the hospital thinking she was having a heart attack, it was so intense. She said she was put on a machine to monitor her heart, just to make sure it was not a heart attack. (we covered chest pains and signs of a heart attack in the last chapter).

Both myself and other widows, found it hard to be around certain types of personalities. I don't know how, but I came up with a name for these ... 'clangers'. Because there was something about them that was loud and big and intense, and I did not trust myself to stay composed around them. It was like they were 'clanging' around me. It was an uncomfortable noise, both inside and outside of me.

Clangers would be high-energy people, often quite animated and loud. The irony here ... that was me prior to all this. So in effect, I could not be around the type of person I used to be! It made no sense, but as I have said, not much did.

Grief changes your perception of things and it makes you feel so unlike yourself. I could not believe how swamped I felt by the energy of these people, it just overwhelmed me and created an anxiety response in me. The thought of getting stuck, feeling trapped in a clanging interaction was unbearable. I did not trust myself to be around them and I just had to get out of there, especially if they were another type I lumped in this category, a person who was particularly abrasive, blunt, opinionated or abrupt.

Just the thought of these interactions was extremely distressing. I could not explain it but the 'fight or flight' response was strong. The questions and uninvited opinions of others about what had happened, how I was managing, how or what I 'should' feel/do/think/cope/need, I simply did not have the emotional resilience to deal with it. I had to remove myself from these situations, they made me so incredibly uncomfortable. They would 'clang' and I could feel my heart start to race. Sometimes I could be reduced to tears. I just had an overwhelming urge to get out of there. I would say to my friends on occasions, 'can we go, there is a clanger in the room' and we would leave or find a different space to escape to. I remember one uncomfortable occasion, I pulled up in the car park at the shop and saw someone I know go in ahead of me. I did not get out of my car. I wanted to avoid bumping into them so much, because of a previous experience, I just drove to another shop!

This is how my grief played out, the impact it has had on my life, and what I had to go through every day. I felt out of control, and exhausted from the spectrum of emotions that surged and demanded to be let out. You may identify similarities with your grief. I hope it makes you feel less alone and more understood.

On reflection, I think the main reason for the anxiety around people is due to the unknown reaction they are going to have to your loss and grief. Everyone I have spoken to said they learned very quickly that a lot of people are uncomfortable around a griever because they don't know what to say and how to act. They clam up and avoid you, or just ramble on and let anything fall out of their mouths without running through a filter. This only has to happen once or twice for you to become very aware that not all people know how to deal with your grief, and it is awful being on the receiving end of that.

They may know our situation but have no idea of what it feels like to be *actually living it.*

And it is pretty uncomfortable for us, too, just sayin'.

How Did I Manage?

So how to cope with these sensations when they arise and not let them lead to a full-blown meltdown? It comes back to having some strategies and some boundaries to look after yourself.

I was explaining to a friend about how this anxiety thing kept happening and I would get emotional and cry. She had been going through her own health journey and told me she would cry whenever she went to the doctor's surgery because it was always a really horrible experience. Her advice to me was that she just accepted that when she went to see the doctor, she would cry, and if on an occasion she did not cry, that was a bonus.

So that became my new strategy. If I go out in public, I might cry and get anxious. If I don't, well that is a bonus. I shared this 'ownership' of my new existence on social media, and it actually helped me reduce the anxiety. I was ok with this, and if anyone saw me in public, well, they would have to be ok with it, too. Instead of getting anxious about getting anxious, I just accepted I might, and suddenly, I was managing it much better, and the intensity became less and less.

I felt like I had regained some control over my life. When your grief is overwhelming and you feel you need to be or act a certain way, try surrendering to the wave of emotion instead of fighting it. That might be something helpful for you.

Friends might ask you to have dinner with them and offer to pick you up. See how you feel about that. You might be ok to go with that arrangement. I enjoyed the company but the thought of not being able to leave if and when I wanted would cause that anxiety to start welling up inside me.

Whenever friends invited me out, I would always tell them I would meet them. I drove there, I could leave if I wanted to, when I wanted to. The thought of being stranded because I had to wait for someone else to leave was too uncomfortable, that in itself would cause an anxiety response in my body. It also made me accountable re alcohol. If I was driving, I could not drink, and I would not run the risk of overindulging.

What about if people visit you at home? They came over to be with you, just chatting away, riding that roller coaster, like good, supportive friends do, and then after a while you suddenly feel really tired or drained, and you don't want to be rude, but you need them to go.

When friends visited me at home, it was ok to be honest and tell them if I was getting tired or I could just say politely that I had had enough and they would hug me, and leave, no offence and no awkwardness.

A couple of weeks after Craig's funeral was my son's 21st birthday. While I wanted to be there for him, the thought of being in a room packed full of people was frightening. I raised this with my social worker and we came up with some strategies for the evening.

For my son's 21st birthday, my mum, my younger son and I took an Uber because carparking would be an issue at the venue. I had organised with my son, the 21-year-old, to leave after speeches, found out where the bathroom was so if I needed to go 'hide' I knew where to go and had a planned exit strategy if I got overwhelmed, which was knowing we could call for an Uber that would be there within minutes!

Is the date you are planning to return to work creeping up on you? How are you feeling about going back to work? Do you feel ready or has it become necessary, as you have used up all your leave entitlements? I thought it was time to try and ease back in after a couple of months off. I was riddled with anxiety and it was frightening. The saying goes 'I could do my job standing on my head with my eyes closed', yet the thought of being in front of people was terrifying. And these people are not in the least terrifying, a lovely bunch and like family to me, so it just did not make sense to be anxious, but I was and it made me doubt my ability to function.

And this was just not ok and I realised I needed a plan if I was going to go back to work.

Before launching full pelt into classes, I decided to go with the idea that was suggested, a morning tea the week before classes commenced so I could see my clients in a casual setting beforehand. They could come and have a cuppa and say hello, get the condolences, hugs and emotions out of the way. Then when I went in to do a class, it was just business as usual, and we could get on with it. When I told my social worker my plan, he said 'ah yes, Exposure Therapy' and my response was with amusement, 'what? Of course, it can't just be morning tea, it has to have a name!'

This was the best decision – yes morning tea was a little emotional for some of my clients and I, but things went smoothly when we got back into our routine. It was much better than just turning up to run a class after a couple of months off, where as you would expect, everyone wants to check in and see if you are ok and hug you, and as you begin, all eyes are on you and you are an overwhelmed, emotional wreck.

I slowly built my workload up from 1 class per day, to my full schedule over a period of 3-4 weeks. I was surprised that after one 45 minute class, I was exhausted. I had no idea that being 'on' for that period of time could be so draining. It felt bizarre, but it was how things were, and I had to adjust and accept this was part of my new normal.

As my days became filled with my schedule of classes, I had to put boundaries in place to manage my energy and my emotional resilience. I could not believe I was still feeling so tired and the 'fight or flight response' that kicked in after classes. I would quickly pack up after and excuse myself saying I had an 'appointment' or a 'phone call'. It sounded better than saying 'sorry, guys I gotta go … I am drained. I am feeling emotional, and anxious and I might lose it if I don't get out of here'.

Or worse, just have a meltdown in front of everyone.

I used the 'appointment' and 'phone call' excuse to escape uncomfortable situations before I started to unravel before their eyes. These 'appointments' could just be getting in my car, closing my eyes and breathing. Or finding a quiet spot to have a coffee and just press the pause button.

Other times it was all about getting back home to be with my pets and shut myself off from the world.

Grief is unpredictable. Music, a certain smell, environment, tv shows, feeling a wave of emotion or noticing you are becoming anxious and fighting it may cause you to feel like you are going to 'lose it'.

Accept this is who you are, for now, and own this new version of yourself. Tell your grief you will call the shots but accept that some days are just harder. I missed Craig terribly on these days. *Everything* feels hard and it is just awful. Then other days feel easier, and I could say I was having a 'better day'. You may feel emotional, but if you accept this is going to happen, it is a little easier to 'ride the wave' and keep it manageable. You may find that it settles down and you don't have the extreme reactions as much.

Jodie's Tips:

» Give yourself permission to go with the flow of emotions and take the pressure off yourself to act like you are ok. You are not ok, and that is ok. Waves of emotion hit you out of the blue. You will be talking just fine then suddenly your voice shakes and a lump forms in your throat and you start to cry, and then it washes over you, subsides and you are able to speak normally again.

» Just go with it, don't fight it, talk through it and accept this may happen from time to time. If people see you are managing it, it exposes them to the reality of what you are going through and that if you are 'riding the wave', they can too.

» Develop strong boundaries to protect your energy and emotional resilience. It is important you put yourself first and take care of you. As I said before, it is exhausting being you, so create an exit strategy for when it is time to leave or if you feel you need some breathing space. 'Appointments' and 'phone calls' worked for me. People will understand you have to go. Be aware of how much of your energy you can give to others and take time out for yourself.

» If you make plans and it feels like it is all too hard on the day or night, don't be scared to cancel. Trust yourself, if it feels like a good idea, go with it, if not, create an alternative plan. Just be honest with your friends and tell them up front that you get tired easily and you may not be up for a long visit or a late night. If you don't feel up to a visit, reschedule.

» Create a plan to return to work. If going straight back to full-time seems impossible, discuss a plan to return part-time and build your time back up. You may be surprised by how emotionally, mentally and physically taxing it is on you.

Getting anxious about getting anxious is probably worse than the anxiety itself. Accept you are not yourself. New emotions are going to come and go, and you have no control over it. The more you try to fight it, the harder it is and the more emotional you become.

Going into things without a plan or a strategy can make everything feel so much harder to deal with.

Exit strategies for removing yourself from uncomfortable situations are helpful and important.

What We Covered

- When getting anxious about getting anxious becomes out of control
- How did I manage?

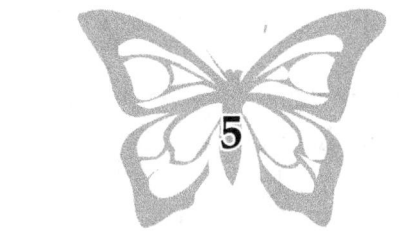

5

Supporting Someone Who Is Grieving

'Everyone can master a grief, but he who has it'
~ William Shakespeare ~

This is a good chapter for the people in your life to read. They may identify with one of the points below, maybe they won't.

But the aim of this chapter is to let them know what they need to know to be there for you. This is about equipping them with what they need, but it might also help you work out how to ask for what you need, too.

This chapter is:

- For the ones who are there, right there in your grief with you, letting you be whatever you are at any given moment.
- For the ones who don't really know what to do or how to be around you but are there, trying their best to support you.
- For the uncomfortable ones who are also there on occasions because it feels like it's the right thing to do.
- For the uncomfortable ones who avoid you.
- For the ones who want to be there but are scared to be around you in case they remind you of your loss.
- For the ones who feel for you, from a distance.
- For the people who just do not know what to say or what to do, so they stay away.

- For those who think grief is something we should not discuss.
- For those that think if you leave someone alone to grieve 'they'll be right'.
- For the people who 'clang' in your life.
- For your community.

It is a helpful guide so you can learn how to get the support you need, and what to do when (not if) someone says unhelpful things to you.

Grief is incredibly uncomfortable for people. Just by saying the word grief, I have observed people's body language change, they look down, shuffle their feet, there is a sharp intake of breath, and an awkward nod.

The intent of this chapter is to bring to awareness to how and what we say and do when we are around someone grieving. This is an important conversation to have. As a society, our attitudes about grief need to change, so we can support people who are grieving better, and know how to reach into them, when they struggle to reach out to us.

People do not always know what to say. They do not always know what to do. For a griever, the sad and harsh reality is these people may avoid them for fear of not knowing how to deal with a loss and how a person grieves, leaving the griever feeling abandoned, isolated and alone.

Some widows felt crushed by things that were said to them, that some people avoided them, some said they did not feel comfortable talking about their loss because of past experiences with unhelpful comments. Others said that they knew people meant well and were trying to be nice, but they made allowances for the awkwardness when things did not always come across the way someone had intended, one widow saying 'I am a forgiving person. I recognise they are uncomfortable'.

When You Know Better, You Can Do Better

I write this chapter with full disclosure – I know I have done or said some unhelpful things in the past. I have been a WIP (well-intentioned person). While I cannot articulate exactly what I said and to whom, I just know I am guilty of saying the wrong thing. I would have thought it was the most appropriate thing to say to someone who was grieving at that time because I had heard (programming) other people say these things. I just know I would have said something similar. I thought I was offering some form of comfort.

Hindsight and my own personal experience with this tells me I am 100% certain I did not.

Because when you are on the receiving end of these comments, when you are being told these things, it is a completely different and often awkward and awful experience. But I am a big believer in 'when you know better, you can do better', something I learned from health coaching, so this is the point of this chapter. To learn there are better ways and to try and be open to learning, to get comfortable with being uncomfortable. I started to ask the question 'if you can't cope with my grief, how are you going to cope with your own when it comes and wreaks havoc in your life?' Because if you love, if you care, if you have relationships of any kind, have pets, enjoy a career, you will without a doubt, experience grief.

That is a given.

The Thing I Really Want You to Understand Is This ...

When a person who is grieving talks to you about their loss and they feel like they are not heard, or they are being judged for their feelings or the way their person died, if any unhelpful comment is made, they will see you as unsafe and they will not open up. They start to feel like no one understands and it is not safe to discuss their loss, or grief with anyone. This is not ok. They need to know they are safe to talk about the loss of their person and their feelings, whatever and however they feel.

And when you lose your person, people do care and they do want to pass on their condolences. But unfortunately, there are a number of things that are said to many widows and widowers that while 'well-intentioned' are really not helpful. These phrases and condolences may sound like an appropriate thing to say to offer comfort but as they are released from their mouth without running through a filter, words can land on the ears of the griever as hurtful, insensitive, judgemental and all too often, are not aligned with the feelings the griever is experiencing, or their beliefs.

Other widows and widowers had similar experiences to me, they saw the discomfort and the awkwardness. Some felt abandoned. Some felt the absence of close friends and family who they thought would be there. They did not feel comforted by some people, and they would try to avoid being around them.

All of us have experienced hearing unhelpful comments, feeling hurt, and some of us did feel angry that someone could seemingly be so insensitive. After many months, I started to push back, stating my thoughts on what was said to me in the hope those words would not be uttered so flippantly to another person who was grieving.

Sometimes I felt resentful that I was put in the position of feeling responsible for that person's feelings, when I was fragile, vulnerable and emotionally exhausted. People would say things that I felt were inappropriate and even if I tried to shut it down and change the subject, they didn't get the hint.

It is all too familiar for widows. Some people would keep banging on about their perception of your situation, and you just want to scream at them to shut up, but you don't because you know in about a half an hour, neither one of you is going to feel good about that interaction.

On one occasion somebody said something that did not help, they tried to tell me they knew how I felt. I remember thinking to myself 'uh-oh'. They then went on to tell me about the time they lost someone and compared a completely different type of loss to mine. What they described was not even close. I felt hurt.

And by doing this, this person made it feel unsafe for me to talk about my loss with them. They wanted me to, they were interested, and they cared, but they had no idea that what they just did unintentionally was make it feel so uncomfortable for me to share. They really had no idea how I felt.

The comment felt like a 'slap'. I wanted to yell, 'you have no idea, actually'. Instead, I clammed up. Yet if I was to suggest that what was said hurt, the person who was 'just trying to be nice and supportive' would have felt slighted and unappreciated, or hurt, too.

I am not alone in this type of experience.

What usually happens, when we have voiced how we feel, is another person will quickly jump to defend, saying that people meant well. This happens a lot, because they too, are unable to see it from the griever's perspective. It does not make it any easier though.

I have to say some of us have had so many things said to us that are 'well-intentioned' but have actually hurt or made us feel unsafe enough times that we actually brace ourselves when someone goes to say something … you feel yourself tense up because you just have that previous experience of things not being kind or comforting or even nice.

I want this to be an opportunity for change. This chapter is written to educate and raise awareness, to say just because it is the way it has always been done, does not in fact make it right or ok.

Anymore.

Regurgitated platitudes and stock standard responses are not always helpful.

Of course, I *don't* actually think most people intentionally want to upset a griever any more than they are, but this is why this topic has a whole chapter dedicated to it.

Because it just keeps happening and we are not learning from it. Nothing is really changing.

I want this to change. So do the many widows I spoke with, newly bereaved widows I have come in contact with since, and other clients I now work with who have lost people close to them, too. Many of them thanked me for writing this book. One widow told me 'you are doing what every widow wishes she could do – you must do this!'

I want society to be armed with some tools, some skills to help people help those who are looking to them to be the support they need.

And to be spared these horrible situations.

So as a society, we get better at this.

Let's Look at What Doesn't Help

We will start with unhelpful comments and actions that have been described by people who have *actually* experienced these:

- I know how you feel … This one is a big No. You know how you felt when you experienced a loss. This is all you know. It is that simple. Please ask how we are, don't assume you know.
- They are in a better place … *according to who?* Many widows and widowers believe their person should be right here with them. Today. Unless the griever states this and *absolutely believes that this statement is emotionally true for them*, it really should be avoided.
- It is God's plan or will … this is a very dicey area. If you are speaking to someone who does not share your religious views, is atheist or agnostic, this is completely inappropriate. And also, for your consideration, a griever may wonder what sort of a God would take a person away from their family, whether they believe in, or have a relationship with God or not.
- You will always have your memories … said soon after the person has died – it's not really comforting to hear that at this point, we want our person back, not our memories.

- Any sentence beginning with 'at least ...' Please, just don't. It can diminish the emotions felt by the griever as well as the person who died because it implies there is a silver lining to this horrible experience. And to a grieving widow or family at this time, maybe there really isn't.
- Everything happens for a reason ... this is up there with God's plan. What possible reason could there be to justify an accident, an illness, a health episode, a death? This can feel cold, uncaring and mean to a person grieving a loss.
- Passing judgement or commenting *on the lifestyle choices* of the person who died, like it is 'justified' they died because of their choices? This really does not help or offer any comfort at all. It is not what a grieving family want to hear.
- And following that up with *'so sorry I didn't get you that book on how s/he could have healed themselves* ... you might imagine this did not go over well.
- They had a good innings ... quite a common one. But this person was more than their age to their family, and they are dearly missed. It offers little comfort to a griever, it may feel dismissive and insensitive.

- You are so strong, just be strong, stay strong or *anything* relating to the word strong ... how a griever appears on the surface has little to do with how they feel on the inside. Don't assume they act from a place of strength. They may be screaming on the inside!
- Telling them, 'it will take time' ... Time without action won't really help the griever move forward toward healing. What the griever does with the time to deal with their grief is what will help them.
- Telling them, *'it has been long enough'* and *'get over it'* or *'aren't you over that yet?'* ... there is no deadline, no calendar date, no magic pill to take to move forward from a loss. This is not like catching a cold that you get over.
- You will meet someone else/there are plenty more fish in the sea ... telling someone to replace their loss with a new relationship can be insensitive and inappropriate. Some widows felt angry when told this. It hurts. We don't want to hear that. We want our husbands. We feel like part of us is missing.
- You just need to keep busy ... until? And then what? Distraction will only work short term. Widows said they often found nights harder because being distracted, keeping busy during the day meant their painful emotions surfaced

when they were no longer distracted. They may also start engaging in activities that offer short-term relief but offer little help to moving beyond the pain of their loss ... bingeing on Netflix, alcoholism, workaholism, online gambling or shopping, exercise, drugs, sex, food, isolation. And anything in excess is not healthy.
- Telling a griever how they should or should not feel, or how to grieve ... everyone grieves in their own way. How you grieve may not be how another does, so respect that everyone will react differently to each loss.
- Offering to take a widower to a 'massage parlour' ... incredibly insensitive and inappropriate. Very hurtful, and in their words, you could not get it more wrong.
- Telling a griever they are jealous of others because of the emotions they are experiencing as they grieve the loss of future life events, the unmet hopes, dreams and expectations, due to losing their loved one. It is not jealousy, it is *grief* – the emotions that arise when a griever realises their person will not be there to share in future life events like births, weddings, graduations, retirement etc.

- Not acknowledging the loss … grievers want to talk about their loved one and hear their name. Avoiding talking about their loved one or avoiding it if it comes up can just plain hurt, it feels like you don't care.
- Tilted head and 'sad pity face' … this gets tiresome. A griever does not want your pity. They want and need your friendship and support.
- Making light-hearted jokes about how long the queue is at the funeral … comparing it to lining up to get into a packed out store that is having a sale, felt so distasteful and disrespectful.
- Crossing the street or turning your trolley up another aisle at the shop to avoid interacting … just hurts. We see you. This can bring up feelings of abandonment and isolation and that no one cares.
- Disappearing when you said you would be there … it can feel like abandonment and it can hurt. It raises the question 'did you really mean it when you said you would be there, or was that just a 'well-intentioned' comment you made in the moment?' It might make a griever feel isolated. They notice your absence.
- Asking lots of questions about *'how will you cope? what will you do? where will you go?'* they may not even know what day it is. Feeling overwhelmed with funeral arrangements and

dealing with the business side of losing a spouse is incredibly stressful, emotional and draining without feeling like they need to have all the answers.
- Saying that their person who died *'would not want them to give up and go live life'* … this can offer little comfort to a griever. You don't know what the person who died wanted. And the griever is going to feel whatever it is they feel, no matter what you tell them. It can make them feel unheard and that their emotions are invalid.
- Make jokes or insensitive comments about suicide, including questions like *'did you know they would do that?'* As it was stated, if anyone had any reason to suspect their spouse would take their own life, would they have left them alone? Please just stop and think about what you are going to say before you say it. This is an extremely difficult time of many conflicting emotions, feeling judged is not needed.
- Brushing the griever off … we get that you might feel uncomfortable, but the griever is feeling pretty uncomfortable too. Try showing a little compassion and empathy.
- Saying or believing the griever needs time alone to grieve. They may already feel isolated so making assumptions about them needing alone time may be your way of dealing with grief but not necessarily what *they* need.

- Telling the griever that you did not like their spouse or comment on how you felt about their relationship … no matter what your intentions are for this, probably best to keep your opinions to yourself. They may be having a hard time processing their own emotions without having to take on board other people's.
- Platitudes – dull, trite, lacking substance, overused cliché, words with little thought. No, I am not being mean, this is literally the definition. And these can make the griever feel like their emotions are invalid and devalues the life of the person who has died. They can sound empty, uncaring and insensitive.
- Comparing your loss to theirs. *Any* loss. All grief is experienced 100%. All loss is loss. No loss is greater or worse or harder to grieve. One person's grief does not and should not negate the grief of another. It is not a competition.
- One person, so many relationships, and all unique. One man may have died, but he was a husband, a father, a son, a son-in-law, a brother, an uncle, a brother-in-law, a nephew, a friend, a good mate, a boss or a co-worker, a mentor and a neighbour. And all the people that were in his life, who had these relationships with him will be grieving their own unique loss. In their own way.

This is a list of *actual* things shared with me from other grievers, widows and widowers, and how it made them feel. I have used their words to describe the emotions. Some of these were common amongst the group. Some were unique to their particular circumstance.

Did you feel this was harsh?

Did you have an emotional response in your body when you read these?

Did it feel uncomfortable?

If you answered yes, you may have experienced what it can feel like to hear these comments from a grieving person's perspective. My intention is to bring awareness to how the many phrases and comments, no matter how well-intentioned, re-used over time are not effective and do not always offer comfort. This is a conversation we need to have so we can do this better, so that we can be there for our grieving friends and family in a way that makes them feel heard, supported and even understood.

How Do We Handle These?

Once I made up my mind that I was not going to put up with more awful interactions, I found these responses helped me when I used them to reply to people who said insensitive or hurtful things:

'No, that is not my experience/not how I feel/ not what I think/does not align with my situation.'

I answer honestly about how I feel. I don't just brush people off. For example, when asked how I am on any given day I will say exactly how I feel, tell my emotional truth:

- 'I am having a good day, thank you'
- 'I am struggling a bit today, but I am here. Thanks for asking'
- 'I am ok. Putting one foot in front of the other one step at a time'
- 'I am not doing so well at the moment. It is really hard, but I am trying. Thank you for caring'.

I will politely ask someone not to finish an 'at least' sentence … in my experience it has never been a positive outcome. I then follow up an explanation for why I did that.

When people compare losses, now I just say that all losses are grieved 100% and every relationship is unique. We can be grieving but also have empathy for other people experiencing loss, too.

People would tell my 19 year old son to be strong for me and I would quickly refute that he needed to do that. He was also grieving his own loss. The word strong more than annoyed me. I hated being told I was strong or how strong people thought I was. If only people knew how much the opposite of strong I felt, I doubt they would have said it to me. I eventually started saying 'well I don't feel strong, so please don't tell me I am'. I prefer to use emotional resilience to describe how I am managing. I have noticed that I have become more emotionally resilient, but that is largely due to the work I have done to complete my emotional business.

Being told I should 'get on with life and move on' infuriated me. How dare anyone tell me how this should go, especially someone close to me, and only 3 months after my husband's death. I get to choose how I survive and live with this, no one else.

As do you!

I still occasionally pull out the 'appointment' strategy if I feel like I need to extricate myself from a tricky conversation I don't think I need to have. I really don't like being schooled on how someone else thinks I feel or should feel now vs how I am going to feel in 2, 5 or 10 years from now, especially when they have not experienced what I have.

So to make my point, I have never lost a child. How could I possibly know how that would feel? Why would I even try to tell a grieving mother 'I know how you feel' or suggest what she might feel? Or tell her how to 'get on with it'. Just NO.

Unfortunately, I still have these awkward conversations occasionally. And like I said, I am more emotionally resilient these days and try to use these moments as opportunities to change perspectives and shift people's thinking, to skill them up to do things differently in the future with other grievers they may encounter or support.

I am not going to leave you hanging. I know you want to know what could be done differently.

Better.

So, What Is a Better Way?

Here are some helpful ways to respond more sensitively to a person who is grieving, from people who shared what worked for them:

- *Having family and friends around.* This was shared multiple times ... According to many widows, this life event exposes the 'real' family and friends in your life. They show up and they stay, and they stay for the long haul.
- *Just hang out in their grief with them*, as uncomfortable as it might be at times. You may not feel like you are helping, but you really are. You are witnessing and acknowledging their pain and their grief and that is *huge*. Just being there with and for them. Be sure to buckle in for that roller coaster ride. You are doing great! Honestly, you really are!
- *Just listen.* I mentioned we were going to discuss this more in Chapter 5. This is what you need to know about listening ... As one widow said, 'we are not depressed. We are not broken. We don't need fixing. We just want to be heard'.

- In Grief Recovery®, we teach people to say something like this to a griever 'I cannot imagine how … devastating/heartbreaking/painful … this has been for you. Can you tell me about it?' Then let them talk without interruption. If you ask them what happened, let them speak. Do not interrupt. Do not ask questions. Do not judge. And don't fuss around, doing other things while they are trying to speak to you. This is their story to tell. *Just pull up a chair and listen.*
- *Grievers do understand that people don't always know what to say to them* and would rather you just say 'I don't know what to say' than something from that *other* list. One widow shared her story of how a friend she had not been in contact with for some time called and said 'I heard what happened and I don't know what to say, but that isn't a reason not to call'. Perfect!
- *They know there is nothing that will bring their spouse back.* You cannot remind them their loved one is gone … they don't forget. However, it is nice to hear their name so sharing stories about your memories of their spouse can offer comfort. Interestingly, this can be quite helpful for close friends or workmates of the deceased person, too. They sometimes feel they want to remember and talk about the person they lost but find it hard to do with people other than the direct family members.

- *Turning up with some cooked meals to put in the fridge to heat and eat.* This was a common helpful thing that many widows shared. They were grateful they didn't have to think about preparing food, especially the women with young families.
- *People with similar experiences can be a source of comfort to a grieving widow or widower.* People who had experienced losing their loved one to suicide or a terminal illness made grievers who had similar experiences feel safe. They felt safe to be open about their mixed and conflicting feelings, they felt 'heard and understood'. Advice about coping mechanisms and strategies from people who have been through a similar experience can be useful.
- *Lending or gifting them a book, articles, or links to helpful websites and presentations that give the griever some useful information about what they are going through.* Again, 'normalising' their feelings, thoughts and behaviour helps them feel less alone in their grief and that they are not going mad.
- *Invite them to join you for a walk/pedicure/dinner out.* Even if they say 'no', please understand it makes such a difference that you cared enough to ask. You may not know it, but it does. And they may say 'yes' next time.

- *Family and friends and neighbours dropping by or calling/texting to check in.*
- *Some found bereavement groups helpful,* others did not. But you might consider offering to go along to a group with the grieving person you are supporting, if they want to do that. Even offering to give them a lift to their session.
- *Reach into them ... A grieving person may find it hard to ask for help.* Some ladies found when people just turned up and did something practical, like odd jobs around the home, was the most useful and positive help they received. Some took washing away and bought it back or put a load on while they visited. You could offer to take the kids to school or pick them up after. Some people just showed up and mowed the lawn or did some weeding.

I hope by sharing examples of what is unhelpful to a griever and the reasons why makes more sense now. Empathy is about being able to see yourself in the other person's situation.

You may look at this list and think it is not as long as the other list. But what you must understand is these points were raised multiple times, so they were deemed helpful by more people. This is your go-to list for how to support someone who is grieving.

There are so many things that could be said or done instead, and I hope when you look at the list, it helps you feel more comfortable and understand how to support someone who is having a really hard time adjusting to life without their person. You do not need a degree in psychology to talk to someone who is grieving. And you certainly are not expected to have a magic wand to fix the situation.

When you see what could make a difference to someone who feels vulnerable, alone and isolated, just making time to pop in for a cuppa or asking them to join you for a walk could be the thing that makes their day brighter and makes them feel less alone.

By mentioning their spouse, you cannot remind them of their loss (they will never forget) just like you can't say or do anything to take their grief away. But it will help them, in fact it may mean the world to them, to know that you care enough to show up, call or offer to do something to help them during this period where they are experiencing heartbreaking, scary, emotionally challenging days.

Jodie's Tips:

» Head to www.jodie-atkinson.com.au to download the list of what to do and what not do when a person is experiencing grief.

» Listening to the griever. Don't interrupt, ask questions or keep moving around while they are talking to you. This sends the message that you are uncomfortable with their feelings, and they will not see you as safe.

» Offer to do something – remember they may have trouble asking for help or not know what or how to ask you.

» Just showing up, inviting and including them

» Be yourself, you don't need a university degree to be a supportive friend. Be honest about how you feel and even if you are not sure what to do, let them know you are there for them, by continually showing up.

» Do something practical and useful – do the dishes, mow the lawn, take the kids to school, cook up meals for the freezer. This is so helpful and appreciated.

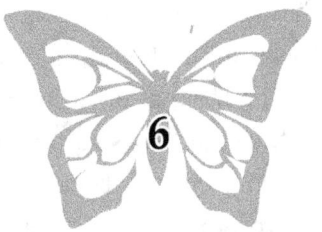

New Existence, New Life, New Identity

'Only people who are capable of loving strongly can also suffer great sorrow, but this same necessity of loving serves to counteract their grief and heals them'

~ Leo Tolstoy ~

Life is different.

The shine has come off everything, and most days feel like you are on a treadmill, just going through the motions. I tried to explain to someone that if I were to describe positive emotions as colour, they are not as vibrant as they used to be. It does not feel like they are experienced at the full velocity at which they were before. Sometimes, it feels like it is just kinda luke warm.

Trying to 'go back' to a life you shared with your person feels like you are constantly falling into the crater they left behind. Creating a new life with new routines and practices, while foreign and at times, messy and scary, can help you establish a smoother transition to this new existence.

Do You Move On or Move Forward?

When I started writing this book I was approaching the 12 month mark since I lost Craig. The first year, for me, was about survival. I just had to get through the year. I plodded along, not making big decisions, sticking to doing work that suited me and establishing a sense of normality. I like the term *moving forward*. Nora McInerney, author and speaker, gives a powerful TED talk on this subject: 'We don't "Move On" from grief. We move forward with it'. It is something I have watched several times, taking something new from it each time. For me, moving forward means carrying the loss of your loved one with you into this new existence, not moving on. Moving on implies that we close a chapter and move on from our loved one. We leave that part of us in the past, like something we should put behind us and forget, and that just does not feel right for me.

Like you, I will carry this loss with me for the rest of my life. It is part of who we are now. And in life, Craig shaped the person I became, as his passing will shape the person I continue to become. He is not someone or something I want to forget about.

The Year Of The Firsts

That first year brings up all the 'firsts ... things you celebrated together – birthdays, Easter, Christmas, anniversaries, special dates of significance. How you choose to honour/celebrate/get through these days will be your choice. And again, there is no right or wrong way.

Some firsts can be hard to think about celebrating or commemorating without your loved one here. Some widows told me that the anticipation of the anniversary days can actually cause more anxiety or be more stressful than the actual day.

And in my experience, it turned out that they were right, especially the anniversary of the death of your person.

Having a plan for how you want to spend those days is a good idea. You can plan something to look forward to rather than the day arriving without you being prepared. What you do on these days is up to you to decide, will be very different and personal for each individual, and again, there is no right or wrong way.

Some days highlight your loss more than others. I was incredibly anxious about my first Christmas without Craig. The thought of being around family, doing the usual Christmas thing, amplified his absence. It felt awful. I did not want to put myself in the position of trying to avoid falling into a giant Craig-sized hole all day. As my sons were spending Christmas with their father, I felt I was able to escape everything Christmas-y. I decided to go away by myself.

Once I had made that decision, I felt a flutter of excitement about taking my dog and booking a pet-friendly cottage an hour out of Adelaide by the beach. There were some people who were concerned about my choice, told me that I should not be alone, but I stuck to my guns, I had made up my mind and I was looking forward to it. I left early Christmas Eve and returned late Boxing Day. It was the most un-Christmas thing I had ever done, and it was just what I needed. I relaxed, read a book, spent a lot of time at the beach, and I started to write ideas for this book.

The second year for me is about stepping back into life and taking action to do more than survive. Professionally, I feel like I know where I am going, focusing on my new work roles.

New Existence

So much change occurs. Waking up each day without your person here in itself is hard enough to come to terms with. The whole world seems different, yet people around you carry on the same, their life seemingly untouched by the tragedy that has claimed yours. I felt that trying to fit myself back into a life that no longer exists made no sense to me and set me up for nothing but more grief and overwhelm.

Sometimes big changes happen soon after. Like moving house. Some widows had a choice, and some did not. Some reasons were the house they lived in was being sold, or it no longer felt like home, they could not afford to stay there, it became too hard to maintain by themselves or there were painful memories associated with the death of their husband.

Some women took very little time off work, others took as much time as they felt they needed, some found they did not have the same level of stability in the workforce and had to keep looking for new positions, some completely changed careers.

When I discovered The Grief Recovery Method®, I decided I was going to become certified to help other people deal with loss and grief and write a book. Those were probably the biggest decisions I made in that first year.

Because I struggled to find the help I was looking for, I wanted to change that, and I wanted to create something to help others experiencing loss to have some sort of tool to navigate their grief. It did not feel right to just try to heal for myself. It felt wrong to walk away from what felt like a gaping hole in grief support that I, and others, had experienced, and let someone else to fall into. I just could not do that.

Like you, I did not choose this life. This is not how it was supposed to be. It takes work, but the way I see it is I can choose to feel ripped off, bitter and angry about that, or accept that I have a choice about what I do from here on. I am 47 years old. I have a lot of time left on this planet, and I want to live again, not just survive, for myself and for Craig. I am still getting to know this version of me as I step into who I am now.

Continuing Bonds

Continuing Bonds was something that my social worker discussed with me, early on in my sessions. This is about recognising the relationship you have with your person has changed but does not have to be ended or forgotten.

Working out a way to do that will look different for everyone. Some people set up foundations in their person's name. Some might take up a sport or hobby their spouse enjoyed as a way of staying connected. Some get tattoos.

Others might plant a tree. It does not matter, it is what feels right for each individual. The important thing is about maintaining a connection, and it should feel positive. If you feel like your connection is painful or negative, there may be some work required toward moving beyond the pain of loss to establish a more positive connection.

Unresolved Grief can get in the way of a positive connection and means a griever might struggle to move forward and experience fond memories of their time with their loved one.

Working Towards Happiness

I had a phone conversation with my mum about some new opportunities that had arisen. Whilst on the phone explaining what I was doing my mum said 'it's good to hear you're happy!' Without thinking, I just blurted out to her 'happy?! What? That's a bit of a stretch'.

She genuinely seemed shocked and concerned when I said I wasn't happy, almost questioning why. I was a little bit sarcastic 'um do I need to remind you what happened a year ago?' I guess she assumed I was 'happy' because I am, well functioning – I have done a lot of work to deal with and heal from my grief – I say yes to more and I am taking steps to rebuild my life.

She said she did not know what to say or do, and apologised, it sounded like she was somehow feeling responsible for my happiness. I said to her that it wasn't up to her or anyone else to make me happy, that is something I have to figure out for myself.

Could it be enough that I have a reasonably positive outlook and feel hopeful for my future, for now, while I work on what happy looks like in my new world?

I said to her 'who knows, maybe it could be a lot of fun working out who I am and what will make me happy now!'

While on the subject of happy, I recall this Facebook post from last year, 2019:

◇◇

30 December 2019

It's almost the end of 2019.

It has been an awful year for many people, struggles, losses and hardship.

I look forward to 2020 with mixed emotions.

This year my life changed.

I am not the same person I was last January. I experienced loss like no other. I lost the man who was my best friend, life partner and husband. A man who took on the role of helping me raise my sons, and unapologetically thought of them as his own. A man of integrity, a big heart, he was kind and a generally all-round good bloke.

He was special. And so so terribly missed every single day.

The impact of that on me, my existence and my family has been devastating, and at times felt catastrophic.

You won't know what I mean unless it has happened to you, you just won't and don't understand. The weirdest things that pop up, the songs, the memories, the events and even just seeing couples interacting, painful reminders of that loss, that feeling of not having him here, you just don't get it, trust me.

It has been the hardest thing, to survive such a loss. It broke me.

I have had to work incredibly hard to get to where I am today.

Through all of this, I have to acknowledge that it hasn't been all completely horrid. The wonderful people who have been there, supporting my family, feeding us, holding space, family, friends and people who have stepped in and said 'I am here' and stuck around when others stepped back. I am so grateful you are in my life.

This year also bought people back into my life, people I lost regular contact with, through distance, time and the changing circles we move in. I am so pleased to have these reconnections and new found relationships through this time of transition. I look forward to seeing them develop and grow in the year ahead. Thank you.

The year also bought me new, unexpected friendships, which I value so much, and am thankful for. I mean taking on all that comes with a grieving person, and quickly becoming a good friend makes for a special person, and I am hanging on to these!

I know how to move forward. I know what I want to do and I know these things because while

I lost Craig, he taught me all I need to know. He gave me what I need to move into a new year, to take opportunities and rebuild my life. I know what I want and I will know when it presents itself. He is my compass and I trust in that. I am doing this, as hard as it is some days. I don't think people realise how exhausting it can still be, getting through a day.

I have lots to look forward to as a new year approaches. I know I am still going to have some bumps in the road, there are still some more 'firsts' to come. I know there will still be times when I struggle.

I am just going to say that I wish you all the best for your 2020.

Working toward Happy.'

New Relationships

For some widows and widowers, the new existence has bought new relationships. One couple met as they attended the same bereavement group and, over time, friendship turned into love. Their story is beautiful, their empathy, compassion and understanding for one another adding another dimension to a special connection. I spoke with them independently and they both shared how they didn't think it could be possible to love two people at once, still feeling love for their respective spouses, but they have discovered it is possible and are looking forward to sharing a future together.

Others have started dating and some have remarried. Others have chosen not to date.

I want you to know that I did not ask any questions about new relationships – all the people I spoke to volunteered this information. I did not ask because in Grief Recovery®, one of the myths of grief we discuss is *replace the loss*. I did not want to imply, even by asking the question, that a way of moving forward is to establish a new relationship.

This is a very personal choice.

For me, I am independent, and finding ways to broaden my social circle, and meeting people who have similar interests. I am the first one in my friendship groups to become widowed, and while I have many wonderful friends, they have their own families and lives. I don't want to rely on them to be my entertainment and be available when I want to do something. I need to take responsibility for my life. I am young, I like to have fun – I am not about to rush out and get a few more cats, stock up on craft supplies and lock myself away from the world.

Financials

This is really important. Unfortunately many widows could find themselves in financial dire straits, in particular younger widows. We can all be guilty of thinking 'it won't happen to me' but the reality is, it can and it might. You need to be thinking about your financial security in the event your spouse dies. Getting some good financial advice about investing, superannuation and other safeguards to access in the event your world shatters apart and you have to adjust to a life without your spouse.

If you are left with some financial security, again, solid financial advice about making that money work for you is crucial. If you are a young widow, you have a long time ahead before retirement and being of age to access your own superannuation or qualifying for some kind of pension, if there is one in the future!

Have you written or updated your will? Organise your power of attorney and even your Advance Care Directive Form. If you have lost your husband, you are all your kids have now. This tragic life event may make you re-evaluate a few things. You may feel these documents are more of a priority than before. Protect your assets, your children's futures and take care of the arrangements in the event you are unable to make decisions for yourself. Organise for your funeral to be paid out of your estate or set up a plan.

Also, if you are on the dating scene, be aware – there are widow social media pages that have reported 'scammers' who have preyed on vulnerable women, and not just online. Yes, as disgusting as it sounds, it happens, and talking about all things loss and grief, a part of raising awareness and having these conversations includes preparing and saving innocent, emotionally vulnerable women from falling victim to these predators.

Family and Friend Dynamics

With the new existence, you may also find that your spouse is not the only loss you experience.

Married friends might start to drop away after a few months. As I discussed this with different people, a number of reasons were raised. One is that the dynamic changes and it feels different to interacting with a couple as opposed to a person who is now no longer part of a couple. And sadly, one thing I heard most repeated was a similar thing experienced by women who are separated or divorced, and that is other women start to see you as a threat – you lost your husband and now you might steal theirs! Yes, it is for real, and it is mentioned here because it came up in discussions. I personally don't understand it, and many of the women I spoke to didn't seem to understand the logic behind this either. But it *is a thing*. Talking it over with others, a possible assumption why this may occur and cause concern or trigger another woman's insecurities could be because a widow may appear to be a damsel in distress who needs to be rescued. Quite often, men may feel they need to help, or provide a solution, fix a problem. This could be why some women think a widow is a perceived threat to her marriage. I don't know why, I just know it exists. And it has done so for a really long time.

You may notice your spouse's friends stop checking in to see how you are. A few widows said this happened, some as soon as only a few weeks after the funeral.

There are other significant losses, too.

Not only do you lose your husband, but you may also lose a family.

Some widows found themselves estranged from their husband's family, with little hope of a continuing relationship. Understanding that everyone grieves in their own way, and the respective relationships each individual has with the person who died, at a time when everyone is grieving, instead of pulling together to support each other, communication ceased and widows felt abandoned and isolated.

There are many reasons this may occur. As confusing and painful as it may be, you might have to acknowledge, that perhaps relationships were not always that strong beforehand, or people tolerated each other for the sake of the deceased person. Maybe your spouse was the glue that held it all together, and now they are no longer here, it is fractured.

Or maybe, sadly, you are part of a painful memory.

This can be incredibly difficult to understand and come to terms with. It raises a lot of complicated emotions. Some members of the family may be struggling to come to terms with their loss and it impacts the other relationships around them. You don't have to bear the brunt of someone else's pain. You can only take responsibility for your own grief and healing. It is not up to you to take responsibility for others.

The thing to remember here, is if this happens to you, realise the importance of establishing your own connection to your spouse, the continuing bonds. Yes, the connection to your spouse's family is *a* connection, but not *the only* connection.

The harsh reality here is that it may never be the same again, and part of your new existence means learning to let go of people who may no longer wish to be a part of your life. This is not always easy. But it might be necessary. You have to look after yourself, too.

I love the analogy of rocks. I learned about this in Grief Recovery®. We carry the weight our grief, toxic relationships and the burden of expectations around with us, like rocks weighing us down. We get to decide to put these rocks down so we do not have to bear the heavy load. The thing is, we have to 'do the work' in order to put the rock down. We might fool ourselves into thinking we have dealt with the crap so we can put it down, only to discover we did not in fact do the work, we just shoved it back in a different spot, it is still there, weighing us down. So, doing the work to put a rock down, and never pick it up again, is important. It means dealing with your emotions, your grief, your 'stuff', getting real and honest, or it potentially remains unresolved grief, which can continue to impact your ability to heal and move forward.

Your new existence, new life and new identity are going to be uniquely yours to design. There is no deadline to work to. You may start to find things that once aligned no longer do, or things you felt passionate about before, are no longer of interest. People may fade away, or show up and continue to show up, and become reliable, stable and unwavering supporters/friends as you navigate this new period of your life. You may have plans and goals you shared with your spouse that you want to pursue as part of your continuing bonds. There are no rules. And no boxes you have to neatly fit yourself into.

Jodie's Tips:

» Don't rush into starting new things.

» Don't make big decisions you might regret later, let the 'fog' settle and when you are thinking more clearly, look at your work and home situation.

» Hang on to valued relationships – family, friends.

» Understand that family and friends may fall away and take responsibility for your capacity for well-being and happiness by doing the work to let them go.

» Establish your own independent and special connection to your loved one, separate to a family connection. Find a way to maintain a relationship with your person that feels right for you, through some form of continuing bond.

» Look at what rocks you are carrying around and decide what ones you can/want to put down.

- » Set yourself up for financial security and find a trusted Financial Adviser to help you with investments and planning for your future.
- » Seek legal advice and write your will, organise your power of attorney and Advance Care Directive Form with directions for the people you are trusting to make decisions on your behalf in the event you are not able to.

What We Covered

- Are we moving on or moving forward?
- Looking at the year of 'firsts'
- Adjusting to a new existence
- Continuing bonds
- Working toward happiness
- New relationships
- Financials
- Changing family and friend dynamics

Final Thoughts

I had no idea my husband would die so young. I had no idea that this life-changing loss and deep, intense grief would be part of my life at the age of 46.

As I think about the journey through this book, I hope that it helps to educate about how grief may show up in our lives, to normalise the thoughts, feelings and behaviour others may experience after they lose their person, to make grief less uncomfortable to talk about and sit with. I hope that we can learn to have more compassion and be more aware and of what is helpful and unhelpful when supporting a grieving person.

As I reflect on everything we've covered over these chapters I do feel a shift from where I was when I started this book.

I have had to work hard in order to move forward, and while I did not rush the healing process, I just knew I needed to do the work, to become emotionally complete and heal from this devastating loss. I dedicated time and action to achieve this and prioritised my emotional and mental health and well-being above everything else. As I grew more resilient, I was able to create the space to include other areas of my life – working my fitness business, which included a new and exciting opportunity, setting up and working with clients in my Grief Recovery® business and giving more attention to my own health and fitness again.

I look to the future with positivity and hope. I am aware

Final Thoughts

I am gaining my sense of identity, not quite the same as before, but I am figuring things out, even though it feels a bit like learning to fly while I build the plane. I feel a sense of purpose and it is such an incredible feeling – to connect with something again.

I am hopeful that we can learn to be more comfortable and accepting of grief in our society. Conversations about how to cope with loss need to be more common.

Let's talk about it and help each other to be more understanding and accepting that, loss – death – is a very real part of life that we will all experience at some point, often more than once, and we could get so much better at being around it, in it and sitting with it if we just had some discussion about it to make it less taboo.

Now we are aware that grief has many forms, when you meet it, you may be in a better position to recognise it when it crashes through the door, kicks off its shoes, and makes its unwelcome presence known. When it unapologetically pushes you until it breaks you, turns life upside down and inside out, to the point you barely recognise yourself.

And how you can learn to *manage* it.

Until you are ready to *deal* with it.

So that you can *heal* from it.

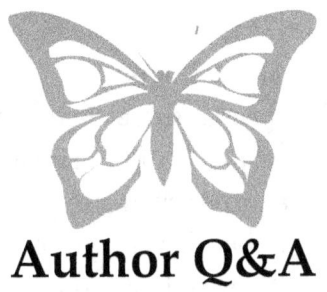

Author Q&A

Why did you write a book about grief?

I certainly did not think my husband would be diagnosed with a terminal illness and die so young. I did not think this would happen to me in my 40's. I was not prepared for this and had no idea how grief would impact my life, because we as a society do not really talk about it.

I had seen other people share their vulnerability online and that helped me feel that I could share my story. I was very open about what I was experiencing in the hope it would help people understand me, but also give permission to others who may be going through a hard time to do the same, and not feel so alone in what feels like a scary new world.

By sharing our experiences and our vulnerability we 'normalise' the behaviour, actions, thoughts and emotions we are dealing with. When you are going through these moments you do wonder if you are losing your sanity and it is incredibly frightening and overwhelming.

Setting boundaries and managing your own expectations about your ability to function might not be so clear and simple for many living with grief. I hope this provides some gentle support and guidance in this really difficult time.

Why are you so passionate about raising awareness about grief?

I was looking for hope when I was at the lowest point. I was getting pretty desperate to find something that would pull me out of my grief, because everywhere I looked, the information was not aligned with what I was searching for. I did not know what I wanted, I just knew I never wanted to be walking out of a counselling session and crying in my car again! I just had this feeling I would know when I found it.

Much of my research into grief support and the experience of others I sought advice from was not helpful. When I discovered The Grief Recovery Method®, I just knew it was what I needed. It was positive, it was a proven evidence-based program, it spoke to me. I just had to provide the very thing I was looking for so others did not feel lost, drowning in grief and feeling no hope.

Loss is something we will all experience in life, but rarely are there real, honest open conversations about what happens when we lose someone or something we love, or if a relationship breaks down. We grieve. It is a normal and natural reaction to loss. Yet we are not equipped to deal with it. We need to talk about it more, make it less uncomfortable and taboo to discuss. We are all going to experience it, at least let's be somewhat prepared for what it might look like.

How do you stay motivated and inspired to do the work you do?

Having someone witness your grief and listen to you process your thoughts and emotions without judgement and providing solutions is so, so important. Knowing that you have been able to access a fantastic resource to help yourself and that you could use that same resource to help others, well, that seemed like a no-brainer for me. I saw an opportunity to help others who were just like me, and I wanted to be there for them as a Grief Recovery Specialist®. I can help someone establish a more positive connection to their loss or overcome the pain of a relationship breakup. I can give them access to something that could be life-changing. That is what this program was for me.

If people have challenges or come up against obstacles around grief what do you say to them to help them persevere?

With grievers, I listen. I let them tell me. I don't judge. I don't lecture. I don't ask lots of questions. Don't fuss around them – this just makes them more uncomfortable and it actually makes the griever feel like you are not safe. Your discomfort about their feelings is showing up, and they sense it.

If people ask me how to best support a person who is grieving, I give them helpful tips, like the ones in this book, ones that grievers themselves have said are useful. I encourage them to just take the pressure off themselves to be something more than who they are and what they feel. Just turn up, hang out with them. Let them talk, laugh, cry, watch a movie. Whatever it is, just be there and let them tell you. And most of all, just listen!

What's your wish for people once they've read your book?

I hope this starts a conversation. Between partners, families, friends. It is one we really need to have.

I hope we can start to be comfortable with grief as it is a normal and natural reaction to loss and while it will look different for everyone, accept it for what it is.

I hope people feel armed with the right information, skills and strategies to see someone in pain and say 'I am here' and hang in there for the long haul.

I hope people who are grieving know there is support out there to help them through this awful time in their life.

I hope people learn that they don't have to live with a painful connection to their loss because they feel it is their only way to stay connected to their person. There is another way.

I hope grievers feel more supported, heard and understood.

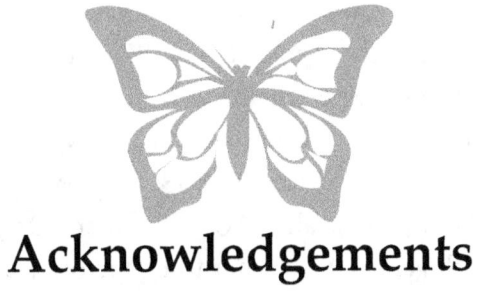

Acknowledgements

I would like to thank the following people for sharing their stories. I hope you know that your valuable contribution to this book is greatly appreciated and I think many will take comfort from your experiences:

Chris, Georgia, USA; Ann, Ottawa, CAN; Pixie, Victoria, AUS; Christel, South Australia, AUS; Jody, Wisconsin, USA; Marietha, South Australia AUS; Jennifer, Oregon, USA; Angela, Michigan, USA; Charlton, Victoria, AUS; Kate, Illinois, USA; Gen, Oregon, USA; Suzy, Yorkshire, UK; Laura, New Jersey, USA; Terri, Florida, USA.

Thank you to my family, my sons, Daniel and Jarrod – love you both more than you know and I thank you for your encouragement and support.

Special mention to my my mum, Gail, for your unwavering support, love ... for having my back, for picking up the pieces, and your constant belief in me to get through the most devastating time in my entire life, even when I did not think I would. I love you. xx

My wonderful friends – you know who you are – you have been there through it all and you are still here today. Thank you for being there through the roller coaster, for saying the right things at the right time. And one of you was always there when I needed you! How did I get so lucky! I love you, guys xx

To Emma Franklin Bell, my writing coach. I am so grateful for your experience, your guidance and support to get the words onto the pages and the message to the world. I honestly don't know how I would have achieved this goal without your wisdom and advice. Thank you so much xx

To my dog, Beau, who is not just a dog. This guy is my best mate. On many occasions he was my reason to get up in the morning, and best thing about coming home. I am not sure what I would have done without him.

To Blaise and the team at Busybird Publishing for helping to craft this book into something really special, holding my hand through the final stages of creation and bringing this to life.

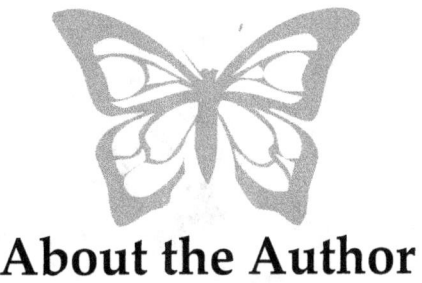

About the Author

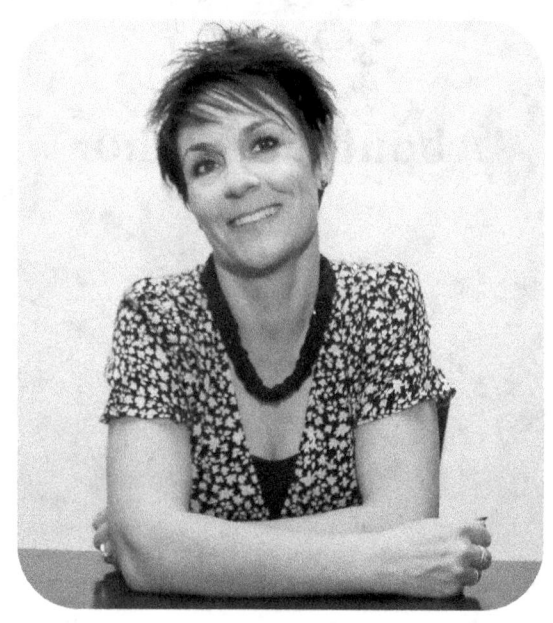

Photo : Rylie Young

About the Author

Jodie Atkinson is a Grief Recovery Specialist®, Personal Trainer, Fitness Instructor and Health Coach, author and speaker.

She is passionate about opening up conversations around loss and grief. Jodie writes (to assist grievers) speaks to grievers within the community and facilitates programs and workshops for individuals and groups to deal with losses of all kinds, with her knowledge and awareness that healing and recovery from significant loss is possible when you take action with time, together.

She intends to continue this conversation with plans for a podcast, so stay tuned!

Resources

- The Hot Young Widows Club Nora McInerney
- Nora McInerney TED talk 'We Don't Move On From Grief, We Move Forward With It'
- https://www.ted.com/talks/nora_mcinerny_we_don_t_move_on_from_grief_we_move_forward_with_it
- https://www.pancare.org.au/
- https://pankind.org.au/

Connect with the Author

- https://jodie-atkinson.com.au/my-book/
- https://jodie-atkinson.com.au/work-with-me/
- https://www.facebook.com/JodieAtkinsonGriefRecoverySpecialist
- Jodie Atkinson (@jodieatkinson_grm) – Instagram photos and videos

www.ingramcontent.com/pod-product-compliance
Lightning Source LLC
Chambersburg PA
CBHW070109120526
44588CB00032B/1399